Women, Girls & Psychotherapy: Reframing Resistance

Women, Girls & Psychotherapy: Reframing Resistance

Carol Gilligan
Annie G. Rogers
Deborah L. Tolman
Editors

Routledge
Taylor & Francis Group
NEW YORK AND LONDON

Women, Girls & Psychotherapy: Reframing Resistance has also been published as *Women & Therapy,* Volume 11, Numbers 3/4 1991.

First published 1991 by

The Haworth Press, Inc., 10 Alice Street, Binghamton, NY 13904-1580

This edition Published 2014 by Routledge
711 Third Avenue, New York, NY 10017
2 Park Square, Milton Park, Abingdon, Oxfordshire OX14 4RN

First issued in paperback 2016

Routledge is an imprint of the Taylor and Francis Group, an informa business

Library of Congress Cataloging-in-Publication Data

Women, girls, & psychotherapy : reframing resistance / Carol Gilligan, Annie G. Rogers, and Deborah L. Tolman, editors.
p. cm.
"Has also been published as Women & therapy, volume 11, numbers 3/4, 1991"–T.p. verso.
ISBN 1-56024-196-9 (h : alk. paper)
1. Adolescent psychotherapy. 2. Resistance (Psychoanalysis) in adolescence. 3. Teenage girls–Mental health. 4. Women–Mental health. 5. Feminist therapy. I. Gilligan, Carol, 1936-. II. Rogers, Annie G. III. Tolman, Deborah L.
[DNLM: 1. Adolescent Psychology. 2. Women–psychology. W1W0433V v. 11 no. 3/4 / WS 463 W872]
RJ503.W66 1991
155.5'33–dc20
DNLM/DLC 91-20845
for Library of Congress CIP

ISBN 13: 978-1-138-98727-2 (pbk)
ISBN 13: 978-1-56024-196-6 (hbk)

CONTENTS

ABOUT THE EDITORS

Carol Gilligan, PhD, is the author of *In a Different Voice*, Professor of Education at Harvard, and a founding member of the Harvard Project on Women's Psychology and Girls' Development–a feminist research collaborative. With her colleagues, she has coauthored and coedited several books presenting the work of the project: *Making Connections*, *Meeting at the Crossroads*, and most recently, *Between Voice and Silence: Women, Girls, Race, and Relationship*.

Annie G. Rogers, PhD, is a developmental and clinical psychologist who is currently on the faculty of the Human Development and Psychology Department at the Harvard Graduate School of Education and a member of the Harvard Project on Women's Psychology and Girls' Development. She is Director of the research study "Telling All One's Heart: A Developmental Study of Sexually Abused Children." She is also the author of *A Shining Affliction: A Story of Harm and Healing in Psychotherapy* (Viking/Penguin). Preparation of this paper was supported by grants from the Lilly Endowment and the Spencer Foundation.

Deborah L. Tolman, EdD, is Research Associate at the Center for Research on Women at Wellesley College, where she directs the Adolescent Sexuality Project. She is currently writing a book based on her research on adolescent girls' experiences of sexuality, *Dilemma of Desire*, to be published by Harvard University Press. Her present research focuses on femininity ideology as a factor in girls' intimate relationships.

Introduction

Carol Gilligan
Annie G. Rogers
Deborah L. Tolman

We bring together papers on adolescent girls in light of the realization that adolescent girls have rarely appeared in feminist discussions of psychotherapy. This absence in the feminist clinical literature parallels the silence about adolescent girls in the literature of developmental psychology. And yet the voices of young women were key to the birth of a psychodynamic understanding of clinical and developmental psychology. In collecting this series of papers, we wish to recover these voices and reframe the clinical understanding of resistance to include both the notion of resistance as a health-sustaining process and the practice of resistance as a political strategy.

Adolescent girls have emerged as key resistance figures in our studies of women's psychological development (Brown, 1989; Gilligan, 1990; Gilligan, Brown, & Rogers, 1990; Rogers and Gilligan, 1988). Conversely, listening to girls as authorities about girls' experience has transformed our understanding of resistance. Resistance in clinical practice has meant obscuring or burying psychological truths or avoiding key memories and feelings, and thus has been seen as an impediment to the creation of a working therapeutic relationship. Resistance is considered a particular challenge in clinical work with adolescent girls, who are known as difficult to treat precisely because of the strength of their resistance and their tendency to leave psychotherapy prematurely. We elaborate the concept of resistance by joining girls' struggle to know what they know and speak about their thoughts and feelings. In doing so we acknowledge the difficulty girls face when their knowledge or feelings seem hurtful to other people or disruptive of relationships. Thus the word "resistance" takes on new resonances, picking up the notion of healthy resistance, the capacity of the psyche to resist disease processes, and also the concept of political resistance, the willingness to act on one's own knowledge when such action creates trouble. In reframing resistance as a psychological strength, as potentially healthy and a mark of courage, we draw on the data of our research which show that girls' psychological health in adolescence, like the psychological health of women, depends on their resistance to inauthentic or false relationships.

We felt it critically important to include voices of girls and women from different races, classes and sexual orientations in this work on female adolescence. In putting together this collection of papers, we invited women from diverse backgrounds to contribute, and also solicited articles about adolescent girls from a broad range of backgrounds.

We have organized these papers into four sections. We begin with three introductory pieces, "Reframing Resistance," in which we develop our conception of resistance in the practice of psychotherapy and in the theory and literature of developmental psychology. In the second section, "Strategies of Resistance," the authors document both psychologically healthy and unhealthy manifestations of resistance among adolescent girls. In the third section, "The Centrality of Relationships," the authors explore ways in which connections between women and girls can both strengthen and impede adolescent girls' efforts at resisting false relationships. In the final section, "Notes from the Underground," the authors address specific clinical problems presented by adolescent girls and suggest new ways of understanding these problems and new approaches to treatment.

We would like to thank Esther Rothblum and Ellen Cole for inspiring and supporting this collection. We would also like to thank Kathryn Geismar, Amy Grillo, Sarah Hanson, Kate O'Neill, and Lisa Machoian for their careful assistance in the editorial work on this volume, and to thank Kate O'Neill for her cover design.

REFERENCES

Brown, L. (1989). *Narratives of relationship: The development of a care orientation in girls 7 to 16.* Unpublished doctoral dissertation, Harvard University.

Gilligan, C. (1990). Joining the resistance: Psychology, politics, girls and women. *Michigan Quarterly Review, 24*(4), 501-536.

Gilligan, C., Brown, L., & Rogers, A. (1990). Psyche embedded:A place for body, relationships, and culture in personality theory. In A. Rabin et al. (Eds.), *Studying persons and lives.* New York: Springer.

Rogers, A., & Gilligan, C. (1988). *Translating the language of adolescent girls: Themes of moral voice and stages of ego development.* (Monograph No. 6). Cambridge, MA: The Center for the Study of Gender, Education, and Human Development, Harvard University.

SECTION I: REFRAMING RESISTANCE

Women's Psychological Development: Implications for Psychotherapy[1]

Carol Gilligan

I. REVISION

In Jamaica Kincaid's coming-of-age novel, *Annie John* (1985), Annie tells two stories about her development. In the first, which opens the novel and begins at age ten, she speaks of living in a flow of relationship which seems endless until one day, in the year she turns twelve, it suddenly stops. Her mother says that they can no longer wear dresses cut from the same cloth, that one day Annie will have her own house, and that she may choose another way. The

Carol Gilligan, PhD, is the author of *In a different voice: Psychological theory and women's development.* She is one of the founding members of the collaborative Harvard Project on the Psychology of Women and the Development of Girls and is Professor in the Human Development and Psychology Program at the Harvard Graduate School of Education. Her most recent publication, "Joining the resistance: Psychology, politics, girls and women," appears in the *Michigan Quarterly Review.* Preparation for this paper was supported by grants from the Cleveland Foundation, the Spencer Foundation, the Lilly Endowment, and the George Gund Foundation.

second story ends the novel. Annie, now seventeen and about to leave Antigua for England, tells the canonical story of human development–beginning at birth rather than age ten and chronicling a seemingly inexorable process of physical growth and psychological separation. But she tells it as a story of hypocrisy and betrayal:

> The bitter thing about it is that they have stayed the same and it is I who have changed, so that all the things I used to be and all the things I used to feel are as false as the teeth in my father's head. . . . So now I, too, have hypocrisy, and breasts (small ones), and hair growing in the appropriate places, and sharp eyes, and I have made a vow never to be fooled again. (p. 133)

Kincaid's coming-of-age novel, in tracing this transformation, shows how a girl's seemingly ordinary yet intensely pleasurable life of relationship turns into a story about betrayal.

Maxine Hong Kingston, in her autobiographical novel, *The Woman Warrior* (1977), portrays a girl's struggle with ways of seeing until finally her "child-sight" disappears: "Now colors are fewer and gentler; smells are antiseptic." And yet, "the throat pain [of childhood] always returns . . . unless I tell what I think" (p. 206). As she reached adolescence, she tried to tell her mother "the true things about me" so that "she–and the world–would become more like me, and I would never be alone again" (pp. 197-98). Leaving home, however, she learned to see the world logically. "Logic," she explains,

> the new way of seeing. I learned to think that mysteries are for explanation. I enjoy the simplicity. Concrete pours out of my mouth to cover the forests with freeways and sidewalks. (p. 204)

I am in a room filled with thirteen-year-old girls–the eighth grade of the Laurel School in Cleveland. Portraits of women hang on the walls, looking down decorously at the sprawl of girls, backpacks, sweaters. The five-year study of girls' development which these girls have been part of has ended, and I want to know how they want to be involved, now that we are writing about this work and presenting it in public.[2] A consensus silently forms and Zoe speaks: "We want you to tell them everything we said, and we want our names in the book." We begin to talk about the details, and Paula raises her hand. "When we were in fourth grade, we were stupid," she says. I say it would never have occurred to me to use the word "stupid" to describe them as fourth graders, since what impressed me most when they were nine was how much they knew. "I mean," Paula corrects herself, "when we were in fourth grade, we were honest."

Adrienne Rich (1979) writes about re-vision as an act of survival for women:

> Until we can understand the assumptions in which we are drenched we cannot know ourselves. And this drive to self-knowledge, for women, is more than a search for identity: it is part of our refusal of the self-destructiveness of male-dominated society. (p. 35)

Writing as re-vision–the subject of Rich's essay–becomes an act of political resistance, offering writers in particular "the challenge and promise of a whole new psychic geography to be explored."

But an exploration of the landscape of women's psychology reveals a resistance of a different sort: a revision which covers over the world of girls' childhood, as girls, coming-of-age, name the relational life they have lived, often most intensely with their mothers, as "false," or "illogical," or "stupid." This act of revision washes away the grounds of girls' feelings and thoughts and undermines the transformatory potential which lies in women's development by leaving girls-turning-into-women with the sense that their feelings are groundless, their thoughts are about nothing real, what they experienced never happened, or at the time they could not understand it.

As girls at adolescence revise the story of their childhood, however, they draw attention to a relational crisis which is at the center of women's development–a crisis which has generally been seen retrospectively.[3] In conversations between girls and women, this relational struggle tends to stir when the subject turns to knowing and not knowing. I begin with three examples taken from different school settings.

II. KNOWING AND NOT KNOWING

I am sitting on a sofa in a large room – the vacant office of a school administrator. Gail sits in a comfortable chair to one side and speaks about "it" – the "problem" which is standing in her way and rendering her helpless, unable to affect her situation or "achieve anywhere near my potential."[4] I am curious about "it" and I wonder if Gail is curious as well. She says, "I don't know." She does not know whether she will "ever understand what the problem was," but she "hope[s] that someday it will be gone and I will be happy." I ask, "How will it go away?" Gail says, "I don't know." I ask, "Are you curious?" Gail says, "I don't know." She feels that she has come up against "this big wall."

Yet at the end, after I have thanked Gail for taking part again in the study and wished her well until the following year, she turns to me and says, "Maybe someday I will draw it." It seems that Gail knows what "it" looks like. What color would she make it? "Kind of deep ivory." What shape? "A giant block of ice, this tall . . . very thick. A cube standing in front of me." Gail says that she could melt it but that she would "have to use very high temperatures."

The phrase "I don't know" signalled dissociation: Gail's separation of herself from knowing what in another sense she knows. Her knowledge clearly involves strong feelings which seem to have been stopped or frozen. Bringing me back to the subject of "it," Gail says that she could undo the disconnection, but that to take down the wall of ice separating her from her feelings would require "very high temperatures" – a melting of ice into water, suggesting tears and anger.

Speaking with Gail, I feel that I am walking an active line of dissociation, being asked in effect if I could stand the intensity of feelings, if I know about anger and sadness which has frozen, or, to switch to a political imagery – I sense that I am making contact with the Underground and being tested to see if I know the password, if I am a member: Am I aware of the inflammatory nature of girls' knowing, and most of all, would I believe Gail if she tells me what she knows or would I – as she sets out to ascertain at the beginning of our next year's conversation – agree with those people who say – as Gail says to me – "teenage girls don't know what they think." It is crucial for Gail to determine my position since her mother seemed to think that Gail's feelings were not hurt by her stepfather's verbal lashings (see Gilligan, 1990b).

* * *

It is early in the morning in the middle of winter, and I am sitting with Sheila in a quiet room in the coeducational school she is attending. Outside the window, light spreads across fields of snow. Inside it is dim; we have lit a lamp and I begin with my first question. "Looking back over the past year, what stands out for you?" It is the third year of the study, and Sheila, now sixteen, says that all her relationships have changed. They "used to be stable and long-lasting, and they are very unstable now." She dates this upheaval to the betrayal of a confidence by a girl she had thought her best friend. Since then, she has "gotten very close and in insane arguments with people, and so relationships go to more extremes: hot and extremely cold. . . . I have come together and grown apart with a lot of people."

Reflecting on these changes, Sheila says that she does not "really like myself enough to look out for myself." Stirred by the sadness of this statement, I ask, "Do you really feel that way?" She says, "Yeah. I mean I do look out for myself, but I care about other people I think, more than I care about myself. I don't know." And with this string of self-portraying statements – "I mean I do . . . but I care . . . I think . . . I care . . . I don't know" – Sheila unravels a relational crisis which leaves her feeling disconnected from others, out of touch with the world, and essentially all alone.

Asked about a time when she felt down on herself, Sheila says, "the last five years" – since she was eleven. And she has developed an intricate strategy for protection, taking herself out of relationship for the sake of "relationships" with people whom she feels do not know or value her. Lori Stern writes about Sheila as exemplifying girls' puzzling tendency to disavow themselves (see Stern, this volume). Extending Stern's analysis, I wish to focus on Sheila's experience of relational impasse – the logic of which Sheila lays out clearly in the course of the following dialogue between us. Sheila describes an internal conversation between a voice which asks her, "What do you want in relationships?" and another voice which essentially cuts off the question and functions as a kind of internalized back-seat driver. I begin with this voice:

Sheila: There is always that little part jumping up in the back saying, "Hey me, hey me, you are not worth while."

Carol: And why not?

Sheila: Because people have shown it. Because my relationships have proven that.

Carol: How can they show that? How can other people know?

Sheila: Other people say, "It has to be true because you are stupid. You don't know it yourself, you are not even worthwhile to know the truth." Other people must know it.

Carol: Do you believe that?

Sheila: In a way.

Carol: And in another way?

Sheila: In another way, I think I must be smarter because I haven't let them in.

Carol: Ah, so if you haven't let them in, then they can't know.

Sheila: I am safe, right?

Carol: But if you let them in all the way?

Sheila: Then it's not safe. Then if I do something, then I know it's me.

Carol: I see. This way you could always say they don't know the real you.

Sheila: Uh-huh. Sane, isn't it?

Carol: It's a very good hedge. But at the cost [of what you have said you want]. It precludes . . . what you have called "honesty in relationships."

As I question the seemingly unquestionable voice which Sheila heeds but does not believe or agree with, Sheila describes her feelings of helplessness in the face of others whom she has in fact outsmarted, keeping herself safe but at the cost of sacrificing the relationships she wanted.

The previous year, Sheila had created a powerful image of relational crisis in describing her relationship with her boyfriend. Her striking and witty description of standing helplessly in a relationship which is sinking captures her own situation and also the feelings of other girls and women who, like Sheila, are reluctant to say what they clearly know is happening:

> It is like two people standing in a boat that they both know is sinking. I don't want to say anything to you because it will upset you, and you don't want to say anything to me because it will upset you. And we are both standing here in water up to about our ankles, watching it rise, and I don't want to say anything to you, you know.

Girls often use the phrase "I don't know" to cover knowledge, which they believe may be dangerous, and the phrase "you know, correspondingly to discover what it is possible for them to know and still be connected with other people.

* * *

I am sitting with Rosie in the teachers' lounge – a small room on the second floor of her school.[5] A coffee pot, unplugged, sits on the wooden desk, and wooden cross-panes mark off the daylight into even squares. Rosie is fifteen, and she says, "I am confused." She knows the disparities between the way she is and the way her mother wants to see her ("as close to the perfect child") and she also knows the differences between the way she sees her mother and the way her mother wants to be seen by Rosie. Caught between viewpoints, she becomes confused in describing herself:

> When I am describing myself, I am confused. Just really trying to sort everything out and figure out what exactly my viewpoints are. Putting things in order and deciding how to think about things.

Rosie knows she is not the perfect girl whom her ambitious and successful Latina mother imagines – the girl who "gets straight A's and has a social life but still gets home exactly on the dot, on time, and does everything her parents' say, and keeps her room neat." I ask, "Are there girls like that?" Rosie says, "Perhaps, saints." "Do saints have sex," I wonder aloud, thinking of Rosie whose mother has just discovered that she is having sex with her boyfriend. And Rosie begins, "I don't know," but then fills in what has been her solution: "If they want, as long as they don't get caught, as long as nobody knows.

Yet Rosie intensely wants to be known by her mother. Once her mother knows about her sexuality, Rosie says, "I hunted her down and made her talk to me, and it wasn't like a battle or anything. I just wanted to see what she had to say." But Rosie's viewpoints are so radically disruptive of the order of her mother's household that Rosie may wonder whether, by changing her own viewpoint or perhaps arranging things differently, she might be able to repair what otherwise seems an irreparable division: between staying in touch with herself thereby knowing what she is seeing and feeling ("I looked at her little study and bedroom, and they are a mess too") and staying in connection with her mother's way of seeing herself and Rosie. "So," Rosie concludes, "I don't know."

III. A PERSISTENT OBSERVATION

Beginning in the nineteenth century, psychiatrists and psychologists have consistently marked adolescence as a particularly difficult time in women's development – a time when girls "are more liable to suffer" (Henry Maudsley, 1879, cited in Showalter, 1985, p. 130). And among the girls who suffer in adolescence are those who seem most psychologically vital. Elaine Showalter quotes the following passage from Josef Breuer as illustrative:

> Adolescents who are later to become hysterical are for the most part lively, gifted, and full of intellectual interests before they fall ill. Their energy of will is often remarkable. They include girls who get out of bed at night so as secretly to carry out some study that their parents have forbidden for fear of

> their overworking. The capacity for forming sound judgments is certainly not more abundant in them than in other people; but it is rare to find in them simple, dull intellectual inertia or stupidity. (p. 158)

Michelle Fine (1986), studying high school drop outs at the end of the twentieth century, notes that the girls who drop out of inner-city schools – at the time they drop out – are among the least depressed and the brightest. Lively, intelligent, and willful girls at both ends of the century and the social class spectrum thus find themselves in trouble at adolescence.

Anne Petersen (1988), reviewing the literature on adolescence, pulls together a series of findings which provide further evidence that girls are likely to experience psychological problems at this time. Adolescence witnesses a marked increase in episodes of depression, eating disorders, poor body image, suicidal thoughts and gestures, and a fall in girls' sense of self-worth. Petersen's review extends the impressions of clinicians across the century that girls at adolescence experience a kind of psychic constraint or narrowing (Freud, 1905,1933; Horney, 1926; Miller, 1984; Thompson, 1964) and suffer from a range of depressive symptoms, dissociative processes, and "as if" phenomena (Demitrack et al., 1990; Deutsch, 1944; Rutter, 1986).

Epidemiological studies offer further evidence. Elder and Caspi (1990) report that when families are under stress – whether from marital conflict, economic hardship, or fathers going off to war – the children who are most psychologically at risk are boys in childhood and girls at adolescence. Block (1990) reports a sudden drop in girls' resiliency around the age of eleven, with no corresponding finding for boys. Seligman (1991) finds that "girls, at least up to puberty, are more noticeably optimistic than boys," (p. 125) and concludes that "whatever causes the huge difference in depression in adulthood, with women twice as vulnerable as men, it does not have its roots in childhood. Something must happen at or shortly after puberty that causes a flip-flop – and hits girls very hard indeed" (pp. 149-150). And a recent national survey (Greenberg-Lake Analysis Group, 1991) finds that white girls tend to experience a drop in feelings of self-worth around the age of eleven,

Latinas experience a more precipitous drop a few years later – around the beginning of high school – and black girls tend to sustain their feelings of self-worth but at the expense, perhaps, of dissociating themselves from school and disagreeing publicly with their teachers.

Taken together, this evidence suggests that girls face a psychological crisis at the time of adolescence – a crisis to which some girls respond by devaluing themselves and feeling themselves to be worthless, while others disagree publicly and dissociate themselves from institutions which devalue them – in this case, the schools. Both solutions, however, are costly for girls. Yet despite this remarkable convergence of clinical observation, developmental findings, and epidemiological data, pointing repeatedly to a striking asymmetry between girls' and boys' development – and one which has clear implications for preventing suffering and fostering development – this persistent observation of difference has, until recently, remained unexplored and unexplained theoretically (see Brown & Gilligan, 1990b; Gilligan, 1990a; Gilligan, Brown, & Rogers, 1990; Rogers, 1990).

IV. GIRLS

Sounds, touching memory, filtering through theory, collecting, like water slowly filling a basin and then suddenly overflowing or rain falling steadily onto the afternoon streets of childhood – girls' voices, shouting, screaming, whispering, speaking, singing, running up and down the octaves of feelings. And the silence. Faces calm, eyes steady, ears open, girls sitting in a circle and then suddenly rising – like a flock of birds. Taking off and then settling, as if by prearrangement. And yet, nothing has been said, nothing is spoken. Only girls' faces and bodies taking in, registering the tides of daily living, following the drifts of thoughts and feelings, picking up the currents of relationship. I wade in.

It is Tuesday afternoon in the beginning of November – just after Halloween. The Theater, Writing, and Outing Club is meeting for the second year – part of a project designed by three women to learn from girls about girls' experience in the time when childhood turns into adolescence and to offer girls in return our help in sustaining and strengthening their voices, their resistance, their courage and their relationships.[6] Ten girls, ages ten and eleven – three African-American, five European-American, one Asian-American, one with a parent from India – and three women (Annie Rogers and myself – European-American psychologists, and Normi Noel, a Canadian-born actor, theater director and voice teacher) stream into the science room of the public school which the girls are attending. The girls have decided this year to teach us what they know.

Two girls stand side-by-side in the center of the clearing we have created. Two other girls – "their thoughts" – stand behind them. The drama begins. One girl says that she wants to play with the other; the other clearly does not want to. As the two girls face into this relational impasse, their "thoughts" articulate the stream of their consciousness – a brilliant rendering of each girls' thoughts and feelings in response to what is happening between them. Finally, the thoughts take over, and speaking now directly to one another, set into motion feelings and thoughts which initially seemed fixed, unchangeable and settled, and in doing so begin to work out the relational problem.

What girls know about relationships and feelings unfolded steadily through our weekly meetings in the second year of the group. The immediate grasp of psychological processes, the keeping of a watchful eye and open ear constantly tuned to the relational surround which we had observed in girls and heard in interview settings (Brown & Gilligan, 1990b; Gilligan, Brown, & Rogers, 1990), now was dramatized directly for us by girls who seemed to want to leave no question in our minds about the strength of their voices and the depths of their knowing and the intensity of their desire for honest relationships between us. The week Normi introduced neutral masks from Greek theater by demonstrating how a face can mask feelings, each girl, going around one by one in a circle, turned her face into a mask and then named the feelings in the mask and the feelings which the mask was hiding. The feelings masked were feeling "ordinary, nothing special" (covered over by a mask that was "snooty") and feeling angry, not wanting to be with someone, hating someone, being bored (covered over by masks that were "nice, 'smiling" and "interested"). "But Normi," eleven year old Joan says at the end of the exercise, "people always mask their feelings."

Girls' facility in turning their faces into the faces of nice, smiling and interested girls was coupled by their ear for false voices – especially the false voices of women in false relationships. On Halloween, when Annie and I brought pieces of costumes, including angel wings for "someone too good to be true," the girls, putting on the wings, instantly raised their voices to the high-pitched breathiness of good-woman conversation, dramatizing both the persona of the too-good-to-be-true woman and the mechanism of disconnection – the use of voice to cover rather than to convey thoughts and feelings and thus to close rather than to open a channel of connection between people. Separating their voices from the well of feelings and thoughts which lies deep in the body, girls did precise imitations of women's greeting rituals and social gestures and in doing so revealed how well they know the timbre and pitch of false female friendships.

Daily, girls take in evidence from the human world around them – the world which is open for psychological observation all day long, every day, "for free." And in this way, girls often see what is not supposed to be seen and hear what supposedly was unspoken. Like anthropologists, they pick up the culture; like sociologists, they observe race, class and sex differences; like psychologists, they come to know what is happening beneath the surface; like naturalists, they collect their observations, laying them out, sorting them out, discussing them between themselves in an ongoing conversation about relationships and people which goes on, on and off, for much of the day, every day.

Eleven-year-old Stephanie, for example, describes herself as a radio – capable of tuning herself into a range of other people:

> Sometimes I feel I am a radio. On my dial is one [station] that's sad songs, one that's happy songs, one that's sort of no caring songs. . . . And then if I am with Rita, I turn to the happy songs and the giggly songs; when I am with Irene, I turn

> to the sad songs and the real songs. And it's just like, I tune myself in.[7]

This relational capacity may well underlie the psychological resiliency which girls show throughout childhood – an ability to tune themselves into the relational world, to connect with different people.

But girls, living intensely in relationships, often face difficult relational problems. Stephanie explains:

> I totally disagree with the song, "Don't cry out loud." I totally disagree with it. You should tell everybody how you feel, if it won't hurt their feelings, of course. Just like talking to stuffed animals or things; it just helps you get out your pains. . . . And just after you cry enough – like into your bunny's soft tummy, you just start to love them and you really grow to love them.

Stephanie is clear about the nature of the problem: You should tell people how you feel, if it won't hurt their feelings. But her solution is deeply ambiguous. Telling her pains to her stuffed animals, she leaves it unclear as to whether she comes to love the animals or the people from whom she has kept her sadness.

In this light, it was surprising to discover the readiness with which younger girls – seven and eight-year-olds – tell people how they feel, mark relational violations, and openly respond to what is happening in relationships, even when their response leads them to experience painful feelings or cause others to be upset.[8] This relational honesty is vividly caught in Lyn Mikel Brown's (1989) example of Diane, an eight-year-old whistle-blower in the relational world. When Diane is asked about a time when someone was not being listened to, she speaks of her experience at dinner when her brother and sister interrupt her and "steal [her] mother's attention." Diane's solution is to bring a whistle to dinner and to blow the whistle when she is interrupted. Mother, brother, and sister, she reports, suddenly stopped talking and turned to her, at which point she said, "in a normal voice, 'that's much nicer.'" Karin, her classmate, walks out of the room on the second day when the teacher ignores her hand and calls on others "to do all the hard problems." Karin (see Brown, 1989; Brown & Gilligan, 1990b) knows that people seeing her in the hall will think that she is in trouble, but she also knows "I wasn't in trouble. I just couldn't take it. So I guess I just left." Asked if her teacher knows why she left, Karin makes a fine distinction between knowing and listening, saying "She wouldn't listen to me, but I told her, so I guess she knows."

Girls' willingness to voice painful relational realities is rawly evident as eight-year-old Jesse, in Brown's description (see Brown, this volume) tells of the time when she went to play with a friend and the friend had another friend over and they would not play with Jesse. Jesse told her friend that she wasn't having any fun "just sitting there" and that she would go home if they did not play with her, at which point her friend, she reports, said "Just go home." In contrast, Tanya, at thirteen, reveals the treachery which flows from not speaking about painful relational realities. She and another friend backed out of a plan to go to camp with a third girl who was, Tanya says, "supposedly my best friend." When the girl discovers what has happened and asks if she can go to the other camp with them, Tanya says to her, "If you want to; it's up to you," while being perfectly clear that "I didn't want her to come." Tanya feels trapped because "I can't say so. . . . I can't say anything to her. Because she'll be hurt, so I have no idea what to do."

Victoria, at eleven, in the face of such relational treachery, opts for radical isolation – "independence from everyone." Describing her withdrawal from relationships in an effort to stay with her own experience, she is unequivocal in her judgment that what she is doing is harmful: "I try to build, it's kind of bad really to do it, but I try to build a little shield."

* * *

Learning from girls what girls are doing at the time they reach adolescence, I mark the places that are both familiar to me and surprising. And notice the sensations which bring back memories, like the feeling of moving without hesitation and the sound of a voice speaking directly without qualification – the open sounds of voices coming directly from the center of girls' bodies. Picking up from girls the feeling of moving freely in a girl's body, I find myself running with girls as I remember running in childhood.

And listening to girls' voices, I also begin to listen with girls to the voices which they are taking in. Opening their ears to the world, listening in, eavesdropping on the daily conversations, girls take in voices which silence their relational knowledge. And as their experience and their bodies change with adolescence, girls are more apt to discount the experiences of their childhood or to place a cover over their childhood world so that it remains intact. Yet, closing the door on their childhood, girls are in danger of knocking out what are in effect the T-cells of their psychological immune system – their seemingly effortless ability to tune into the relational world. Voices which intentionally or unintentionally interfere with girls' knowing, or encourage girls to silence themselves, keep girls from picking up or bringing out into the open a series of relational violations which they are acutely keyed into, such as not being listened to, being ignored, being left out, being insulted, being criticized, being spoken about meanly, being humiliated or made fun of, being whispered about, being talked about behind one's back, being betrayed by a friend, or being physically overpowered or hurt.

Tanya, at sixteen, writes a letter to Lyn Mikel Brown – the director of the Harvard-Laurel Project – about her feelings in response to a paper which Lyn and I had written (a paper which she and Lyn had discussed together at some length) (see Brown & Gilligan, 1990a, 1990b). She speaks of "a voice inside" her which "has been muffled." She explains, "The voice that stands up for what I believe in has been buried deep inside of me." Tanya wants to be in honest relationship with people. And yet, taking in what she is hearing about perfect girls whom people seem to love and admire, Tanya finds herself paying attention to voices which impede her relational desires. "I do not want the image of a 'perfect girl' to hinder myself from being a truly effective human being," she writes. "Yet, I still want to be nice, and I never want to cause any problems."

When Nina – a gifted writer – turns twelve, the word "nice" spreads through her conversation, covering over a world of feelings, as the word "interesting" covers thoughts.[9] These two words, which gain currency in girls' conversation, dull the human world which girls live in, and the magnitude of this loss is evident in the change in Nina's description of her stories.

At eleven, Nina tells me that she is writing a story about "someone during the Civil War" and making her story "a little bit sad," because when the father goes to war, the girl "is really upset." Nina explains:

> He talks to her before he goes, about how he feels about leaving and that he is just as worried as she is, or more worried and more scared. . . . And, you know, she feels like he's never going to come back, which is possible, but, you know, it's not a fact yet. So she has a very, um, a very strange feeling sometimes.

I ask Nina about this strange feeling, and she offers an extraordinary description of the ways in which feelings layer or cascade, one lying over another or one falling into another like anger lies over sorrow which lies next to shock or surprise, all falling into an ongoing stream of upset feelings, calling forth comfort in the presence of the steady hum of fear and continuing surprise at realizing connection – that "he could feel like this too." Nina says, continuing to describe her story,

> Before he left, she realized that he was not, um, totally powerful, but she didn't, um, feel angry at him for that, but she felt very, um, very sorry, sort of, very sorry for him and very shocked or surprised mainly and still upset that he was leaving. And, um, he was trying to comfort her when he told her about, um, about his, his own fears of going, but really she was just mainly surprised and she hadn't realized that he could feel like this, too . . .

I ask, "Why hadn't she known this?" And Nina continues her precise laying out of people's feelings and thoughts in response to one another – an exquisite, naturalistic psychological narration of change occurring through relationship, which then suddenly comes to a stop, as the father leaves for the war and the girl, responding to his wish that she not make it any harder for him, stops feeling upset or at least stops showing her upset feelings:

> He had always been there for her, you know. She had been, um, she'd been hurt . . . and she had been humiliated because she was a girl. And he always understood her and she was very close to him. . . . Her siblings thought it was really brave of him to do it (enlist] right away, but she knew that, he was, he just, if he waited any longer then he wouldn't be able to do it, he wouldn't have enough courage to do it.
>
> *And how did she know that?*
>
> She knew because of the way he talked to her . . . that he was feeling really scared and upset . . . and he didn't want her to make it any harder or anything. After that, she didn't get so upset, or she didn't show it.

Girls around eleven often come to know their fathers as part of the human world which they take in and listen to, and thus they discover what is often unspoken in this culture: men's humanness – men's vulnerability. Annie Rogers (1990) describes girls' "embodied courage," noticing that voice and body, play and knowledge, tend to be joined in girls prior to adolescence, and that this joining issues forth in a seemingly "ordinary courage" – girls' readiness, in accordance with an old meaning of the word "courage," to "speak one's mind by telling all one's heart" (Rogers, 1990). Courage, however, more often connotes, especially for men, an absence of fear and an overcoming of vulnerability – a psychological and physical disembodiment.

This disconnection is exemplified by the father in Nina's Civil War story as he hurriedly covers over the vulnerability he has exposed, overriding his fear in his determination to do the right thing and enlist in the army. But it also seeps into Nina's stories, so that like the daughter in the story who covers over her feelings so as not to make it any harder, Nina at twelve writes as if she did not know what she knows about people and about psychological processes. In fact, her stories at twelve are less about how people feel than about how things "would feel" if they were "able to see" – like a pen with its cap off.

In one story, a lesson in love is reduced to pure adventure as a girl who,

> is trying to, well, she falls in love with this boy . . . and they have these adventures. It starts when they're at a dance and then when she has to leave, his car gets stolen and then they go to the gang. . . . This group has stolen it . . . and he has to fight one of the guys and then they set off in the car and there's a storm and the car stalls and they have to walk and things like that.

The relational world which Nina previously described is gone, seemingly without leaving a trace. And along with it, Nina, the writer of the Civil War Story, seems to have disappeared. "It's really a good story," she says of her romance adventure, "I can tell. It's a lot better than the ones I wrote a couple of years ago anyway."

Nina's stories about how things would feel if they could see are winning prizes in local story-writing contests, and Nina at twelve dreams of becoming a famous, prize-winning writer or at least winning scholarship money for college. What she loves most – writing and reading – has value in the eyes of other people, and to sell her stories on the open market, she has to pay attention to what others want and value.

Focusing more at age twelve on the value of her stories in the eyes of others than on her own pleasure in writing, which she described at age eleven, Nina seems to have diverted her attention from psychological processes to questions of judgment. Now the people in her stories change inexplicably – shifting from bad to good. For example, in one story "a queen who's really a bad queen gets assassinated on the anniversary of her coronation. But three generations later, she becomes "a beautiful, wonderful queen." Sensing with me that something is missing in this story – some understanding of or even interest in how the queen changes – Nina offers by way of explanation the following observation: "It's just the way memory covers up the bad things."

"Cover up," girls are told as they reach adolescence, daily, in innumerable ways. Cover your body, cover your feelings, cover your relationships, cover your knowing, cover your voice, and perhaps above all, cover desire (see also Debold & Tolman, 1991; Debold, this volume, Tolman, this volume). And the wall that keeps memory from seeping through these covers may be the wall with the sign which labels body, feelings, relationships, knowing, voice and desire as bad.

V. A THEORY OF DEVELOPMENT

If psychological health consists, most simply, of staying in relationship with oneself, with others, and with the world, then psychological problems signify relational crises: losing touch with one's thoughts and feelings, being isolated from others, cut off from reality. The zen of development which makes human growth such a fascinating journey is that relationships which are the channels of growth are also the avenues through which people are psychically wounded. Vulnerability – the opening to experience which is at the heart of development – thus always carries with it the risk of being seriously hurt or diminished, and this play of opening and closing, embodiment and disembodiment, is reflected in the two meanings of the word "courage" (see Rogers, 1990).

The evidence that boys are more likely than girls to suffer psychologically in early childhood whereas girls are more at risk for developing psychological difficulties in adolescence calls for explanation and implies a revision – a new way of speaking about psychological development. This difference, I will suggest, also contains a hope for transformation.

Learning from girls about the relational crisis which girls experience as they approach adolescence – a place where development seems impassable – I offer as a working thesis that adolescence is a comparable time in women's psychological development to early childhood for men. It precipitates a relational crisis which poses an impasse in psychological development, a place where for the sake of relationship (with other people and with the world), one must take oneself out of relationship. Because this separation of self from relationship is psychologically untenable and also essentially confusing (if one is not in one's relationships, then the word "relationships" loses meaning), this division must be resisted and some compromise arrived at.

Freud (1899/1900) suggested as much for boys when he spoke about the "oedipus complex" as a turning point in boys' early childhood and also as the foundation for neurotic suffering and for civilization. The pressure girls are under as they reach adolescence and girls' experience of severe relational crisis similarly marks a turning point or watershed in girls' development. But girls' relationship to the culture is different, and also girls at adolescence are at a very different point in their own development than boys in early childhood – with far more experience of relationships and also perhaps with less incentive to give up relationship as the cost, ironically, of entering society. Consequently, women's psychological development – as others have observed (see Miller, 1986) – is profoundly transformational.

The relational crisis of boys' early childhood and of girls' adolescence is marked by a struggle to stay in relationship – a healthy resistance to disconnections which are psychologically wounding (from the body, from feelings, from relationships, from reality). This struggle takes a variety of forms, but at its center is a resistance to loss – to giving up the reality of relationships for idealizations or, as it is sometimes called, identifications. As young boys are pressured to take on images of heroes, or superheroes, as the grail which inform their quest to inherit their birthright or their manhood, so girls are pressed at adolescence to take on images of perfection as the model of the pure or perfectly good woman: the woman whom everyone will promote and value and want to be with (see Gilligan, 1990a; Brown & Gilligan, 1990b; Jack, in press).

Children's healthy resistance to disconnection – the intense human desire for relationship which now is generally taken as foundational of psychic life – thus tends to lead children into a political struggle. Boys in early childhood resist leaving the comforts and pleasures, as well as the discomforts and pains, of their relational life: They want to stay with the people who have been with them. And girls at adolescence resist leaving the rich relational tapestry of their childhood. This resistance calls into question the prevailing order of social relationships and calls forth counter-pressures to enforce that order in the name, currently, of psychological health, as well as for the sake of civilization.

Thus at the time of early childhood for boys, when masculinity seems in question, and in early adolescence for girls, when femininity seems on the line, a healthy resistance to disconnections which turns into a political struggle comes under pressure to turn into a psychological resistance – that is, a resistance to knowing what is happening and an impulse to cover the struggle.

Here, the differences observed over the century between the times of seemingly heightened vulnerability or openness to growth and wounding in boys' and girls' lives contains a promise of transformation. If girls' can sustain in adolescence a resistance which is more easily overwhelmed in boys' childhood, then women's psychological development will change the prevailing order of relationships. Compared with boys, whose desires for relationship, although strongly felt, tend to be less articulate, more inchoate, more laced with early loss and terror, girls' desires for relationship, leavened through years of childhood experience, tend to be hardier, more easily spoken, better known, more finely textured or differentiated and consequently less frightening although no less painful. Girls' healthy resistance to disconnection which springs up at the edge of adolescence as girls approach a culture of relationships which has been built largely by men thus calls into question what has been accepted as the canonical story of human development: the story which takes separation for granted, the story which seems logical, the story which rejects the possibility of honest or genuine relationship – the revised developmental story which Annie John and the woman warrior and the thirteen year old girls superimpose on the story which comes out of their own experience in childhood.

VI. IMPLICATIONS FOR PSYCHOTHERAPY

In my dream, I am wearing my glasses over my contact lenses. I am literally seeing double, although I do not realize this in the dream. I sit with a woman and remorsefully realize that I have wanted too much in the relationship – that I cannot possibly have what I want. She says, "I cannot offer you myself," and the logic of her statement feels overwhelming. And then – still in the dream – I take off my glasses and suddenly say, "No," because I suddenly know that this is not it – this remorseful wanting of what cannot be given. "No," I say, and then go on to speak the truth of my experience in the relationship. With this, my head suddenly swivels, like an owl's head turning 180 degrees around, and I feel – in the dream – a strong jolt, like a shock, and overwhelmingly dizzy, as if I am seeing double. Only after I wake up do I realize that when I felt dizzy was when I was seeing straight, and that in the dream when I felt I was seeing clearly, I was literally seeing double – wearing two sets of lenses which made it impossible to see straight.

I dream this dream on the first night of the second year of the Theater, Writing, and Outing Club which Annie Rogers, Normi Noel and I have formed with eight girls from the Atrium School. We are in New Hampshire, near Mount Sunapee for the weekend. And I realize the next morning that this work with girls is seeping deeply into my dream life, leading me to re-vision – to a new seeing and naming of my experience; taking me back to the time of adolescence, the time, I realize, when straight-seeing became shocking, surprising really in the manner Nina describes in speaking about the girl in her story; angering and yet, at bottom, somehow more sorrowful. The time when relationships flowed – albeit through some rocky places; the time before voice and vision doubled.

Adolescent girls offer a key to understanding women's psychological development. And they offer some suggestions for preventing and treating psychological suffering. To catch girls in the moment of their revision – at the time just before or around adolescence – is to see a world disappearing: a rich world of relationships which seems so powerful in part because it feels so ordinary. To see this world disappearing while girls are saying that nothing is being lost or at least nothing of value, and to hear one story of love begin to cover and eclipse another until, like the moon in the sun's shadow, the under story glowing faintly red, is to ask the question which is at the heart of therapy and prevention: is this loss necessary, is this suffering and psychic diminution inevitable – a question which ties in with girls' healthy resistance and girls' courage (also see Rogers, 1990).

Then the central paradox of women's – and men's – psychological development becomes opened for re-examination: the taking of oneself out of relationship for the sake of relationships. And the incoherence at the center of this sentence – the dizzying black spot where the word "relationship" loses or changes meaning – then becomes the focus of a new question: what would it mean not to give up relationship?

Heads swirl, dizziness descends, threatening blackness, a voice whispers "take cover." As in speaking with Gail or Sheila or Rosie, I am asking myself the question which leads into the underground: the healthy resistance to disconnection which becomes a political resistance or struggle, which then is under pressure to turn into a psychological resistance: a seeing double, a not knowing.

Because women and girls who resist disconnections are likely to find themselves in therapy – for having gotten themselves into some combination of political and psychological trouble – therapists are in a key position to strengthen healthy resistance and courage, to help women recover lost voices and tell lost stories, and to provide safe houses for the underground. Tuning themselves into the voices of girls in the time before the re-vision, therapists can be good company for women as they return through the passages – going backward now – from a psychological resistance which takes the form of not knowing and covers a series of disconnections, to a political resistance which exposes false relationships and brings relational violations out into the open, to a healthy resistance to disconnection which grants immunity to psychological illness – the resistance which is rooted in wanting and having honest relationships.

ENDNOTES

1. I am most grateful for the support and encouragement of Joan Lipsitz and the Lilly Endowment, the late Lawrence Cremin and the Spencer Foundation, and Wendy Puriefoy and the Boston Foundation. The work described in this paper would not have been possible without grants from the Geraldine Rockefeller Dodge Foundation, the Joseph S. Klingenstein Foundation, the Cleveland Foundation, the Gund Foundation, and Mrs. Marilyn Brachman Hoffman. Lyn Mikel Brown, the director of the Harvard-Laurel Project, and Annie Rogers, the director of the "Strengthening Healthy Resistance and Courage in Girls" project have contributed centrally to my understanding of girls' voices and my thinking about women's psychological development. I wish to thank Lyn and Annie, the other members of the Harvard Project on the Psychology of Women and the Development of Girls – Elizabeth Debold, Judy Dorney, Barbara Miller, Mark Tappan, Jill Taylor, Deborah Tolman and Janie Ward, Sarah Hanson – the project assistant, and all of the girls who have joined with us in this work and taught us about girls' experience.

2. The Harvard Project on the Psychology of Women and the Development of Girls began in the early 1980s to explore a series of questions about women's psychological development by joining women and girls, research and clinical practices, psychology and politics. Over the course of the decade, the Project has conducted a variety of studies, retreats and prevention projects at a range of locations designed to ensure the inclusion of different voices – from girls at Emma Willard School for girls (1981-84); to girls and boys in Boys' and Girls' Clubs in three ethnically different Boston neighborhoods and coeducational public and private schools in and around the city (1984-90); to girls ages six to seventeen at the Laurel School in Cleveland – a project that expanded to include women who as teachers, psychologists, and mothers were involved in teaching girls (1985-90); and beginning in 1989, to more intensive work involving women from the Harvard Project and girls from the Atrium School in Watertown, Massachusetts and from a public school in the vicinity of Boston, as well as other women who as mothers, teachers, psychotherapists, ministers and policy makers have become involved with us in this project.

3. For the relational crisis in women's psychological development, see Gilligan, 1982, and Miller, 1986, 1988. See also Belenky et al. (1986), Gilligan, Lyons, & Hanmer (1990), and the Stone Center Working Papers Series. For a retrospective view of the crisis in girls' lives at adolescence, see Hancock (1990).

4. See Gilligan, 1990b, for a more extensive discussion of Gail's experience.

5. For a fuller discussion of Rosie, see Gilligan, 1990a.

6. The Theater, Writing, and Outing Club is a central part of the project, "Strengthening Healthy Resistance and Courage in Girls." This prevention project is designed to help girls sustain their knowledge of relationships and the clarity of their voices into adolescence through theater and writing exercises created to strengthen and expand the range of girls' voices and girls' relationships and outings designed to encourage girls' active responses to the natural and cultural worlds. The project works centrally through developing healthy relationships between girls and women.

7. Stephanie was interviewed by Dr. Sharry Langdale in 1981, along with nine other eleven-year-old girls, and these interviews contributed substantially to a growing interest in the voices of eleven-year-old girls within the ongoing Harvard Project.

8. My analysis of Diane, Karin, Jesse and Victoria draws heavily on Lyn Mikel Brown's work on girls' narratives of relationships (Brown, 1989, in press, this volume; see also Brown & Gilligan, 1990b).

9. In writing about Nina, I draw on conversations with Annie Rogers with whom I read Nina's interviews, as well as on the insights of Kathryn Geismar, Amy Grillo, Sarah Ingersoll, Kate O'Neill, and Heather Thompson – members of the research group on the "Strengthening Healthy Resistance and Courage in Girls" project.

REFERENCES

Belenky, M., Clinchy, B., Goldberger, N., & Tarule, J. (1986). *Women's ways of knowing: the development of self voice, and mind.* New York: Basic.

Block, J. (1990, October). Ego resilience through time: Antecedents and ramifications. In *Resilience and Psychological health.* Symposium of the Boston Psychoanalynic Society, Boston, MA.

Brown, L. M. (1989). *Narratives of relationship: The developmentof a care voice in girls ages 7 to 16.* Unpublished doctoral dissertation, Harvard University Graduate School of Education, Cambridge, MA.

Brown, L. M. (in press). A problem of vision: The development of voice and relational knowledge in girls ages 7 to 16. *Women's Studies Quarterly.*

Brown, L. M. (1991). Telling a girl's life. *Women & Therapy.*

Brown, L. M., & Gilligan, C. (1990a, August). Listening for self and relational voices: A responsive/resisting reader's guide. In M. Franklin (Chair), *Literary theory as a guide to psychological analysis.* Symposium conducted at the annual meeting of the American Psychological Association, Boston, MA.

Brown, L. M., & Gilligan, C. (1990b). Meeting at the crossroads: The psychology of women and the development of girls. Manuscript submitted for publication.

Debold, E. (1991). The body at play. *Women & Therapy.*

Debold, E., & Tolman, D. (1991, January). Made in whose image? Paper presented at the Ms. Foundation's Fourth Annual Women Managing Wealth Conference, New York.

Demitrack, M., Putnam, F., Brewerton, T., Brandt, H., & Gold, P. (1990). Relation of clinical variables to dissociative phenomena in eating disorders. *The American Journal of Psychiatry, 147*(9), 1184-1188.

Deutsch, H. (1944). *Psychology of women,* Vol. I. New York: Grune & Stratton.

Elder, G., & Caspi, A. (1990). Studying lives in a changing society: Sociological and personological explorations. In A. Rabin, R. Zucker, R. Emmons, & S. Frank (Eds.), *Studying persons and lives* (pp. 226-228). New York: Springer.

Fine, M. (1986). Why urban adolescents drop into and out of public high school. *Teachers College Record, 87*(3), 393-409.

Freud, S. (1899/1900). The interpretation of dreams. In J. Strachey (Ed. and Trans.), *The standard edition of the complete psychological works of Sigmund Freud* (Vols. IV & V). London: Hogarth Press.

Freud, S. (1933). New introductory lectures on psychoanalysis (Lecture XXXIII: Femininity). In J. Strachey (Ed. and Trans.), *The standard edition of the complete psychological works of Sigmund Freud* (Vol. XXII). London: The Hogarth Press.

Freud, S. (1905). Three essays on the theory of sexuality. In J. Strachey (Ed. and Trans.), *The standard edition of the complete psychological works of Sigmund Freud* (Vol. VII). London: The Hogarth Press.

Gilligan, C. (1982). *In a different voice: Psychological theory and women's development.* Cambridge, MA: Harvard University Press.

Gilligan, C. (1990a). Joining the resistance: Psychology, politics, girls and women. *Michigan Quarterly Review, 29*(4), 501-536.

Gilligan, C. (1990b). Teaching Shakespeare's sister: Notes from the underground of female adolescence. In C. Gilligan, N. Lyons, & T. Hanmer (Eds.), *Making connections: The relational worlds of adolescent girls at Emma Willard School* (pp. 6-29). Cambridge, MA: Harvard University Press.

Gilligan, C., Brown, L. M., & Rogers, A. (1990). Psyche embedded: A place for body, relationships, and culture in personality theory. In A. Rabin, R. Zucker, R. Emmons, & S. Frank (Eds.), *Studying persons and lives* (pp. 86-147). New York: Springer.

Gilligan, C., Lyons, N., & Hanmer, T. (Eds.). (1990). *Making connections: The relational worlds of adolescent girls at Emma Willard School.* Cambridge, MA: Harvard University Press.

Greenberg-Lake Analysis Group Inc. (1991, January). Shortchanging girls, shortchanging America: A nationwide poll to assess self esteem, educational experiences, interest in math and science, and career aspirations of girls and boys ages 9-15. (Available from The American Association of University Women, 515 Second Street NE, Washington, DC 20002).

Hancock, E. (1989). *The girl within: A groundbreaking new approach to female identity.* New York: Fawcett Columbia.

Horney, K. (1926). The flight from womanhood. *International Journal of Psychoanalysis,* 7, 324-339.

Jack, D. (in press). *Silencing the self: depression and women.* Cambridge, MA: Harvard University Press.

Kincaid, J. (1985). *Annie John.* New York: Farrar Straus Giroux.

Kingston, M. H. (1977). *The Woman Warrior.* New York: Alfred A. Knopf.

Miller, J. B. (1984). The development of women's sense of self. *Work in Progress, No. 12.* Wellesley, MA: Stone Center Working Papers Series.

Miller, J. B. (1986). *Toward a New Psychology of Women* (second edition). Boston: Beacon.

Miller, J. B. (1988). Connections, disconnections and violations. *Work in Progress, No. 33.* Wellesley, MA: Stone Center Working Papers Series.

Petersen, A. (1988). Adolescent development. *Annual Review of Psychology, 39,* 583-607.

Rich, A. (1979). *On lies, secrets, and silence: Selected prose, 1966-1978.* New York: Norton.

Rogers, A. (1990). The development of courage in girls and women. Unpublished manuscript, Harvard University, Project on the Psychology of Women and the Development of Girls, Cambridge, MA.

Rogers, A. (1991). A feminist poetics of psychotherapy. *Women & Therapy.*

Rutter, M. (1986). The developmental psychopathology of depression: Issues and

perspectives. In M. Rutter, C. Izzard, & P. Read (Eds.), *Depression in young people: Developmental and clinical perspectives.* New York: Guilford Press.
Seligman, M. E. P. (1991). *Learned optimism.* New York: Random House.
Showalter, E. (1985). *The Female Malady.* New York: Penguin.
Stone Center Working Papers Series. *Work in Progress.* Wellesley, MA: Wellesley College.
Stern, Lori. (1991). Disavowing the self in female adolescence. *Women & Therapy.*
Thompson, C. (1964). *Interpersonal psychoanalysis.* New York: Basic.
Tolman, D. (1991). Adolescent girls, women and sexuality: Discerning dilemmas of desire. *Women & Therapy.*

A Feminist Poetics of Psychotherapy

Annie G. Rogers

WRITING: AGAINST THE ANGEL IN THE CONSULTING ROOM

In "Professions for Women" Virginia Woolf (1921/1944) describes her struggle to write against "the Angel in the House."

> It was she who bothered me and wasted my time and so tormented me that at last I killed her. . . . She was intensively sympathetic. She was immensely charming. She was utterly unselfish. She sacrificed herself daily. If there was a chicken, she took the leg; if there was a draught, she sat in it – in short she was so constituted that she never had a mind of her own or a wish of her own, but preferred always to sympathize with the minds and wishes of others. Above all, I need not say it, she was pure. . . . And when I came to write I encountered her with the very first words. The shadow of her wings fell on my page; I heard the rustling of her skirts in the room . . . she slipped behind me and whispered, "My dear, you are a young woman. You are writing about a book that has been written by a man. Be sympathetic; be tender; flatter; deceive; use all the

---

Annie G. Rogers, PhD, is a developmental and clinical psychologist who is currently on the faculty of the Human Development and Psychology Department at the Harvard Graduate School of Education and a member of the Harvard Project on the Psychology of Women and the Development of Girls. She is the Director of the research study and prevention project: "Strengthening Healthy Resistance and Courage in Girls." Her paper is a condensed chapter from her unpublished book: *Two Playing: A Feminist Poetics of Psychotherapy.* Preparation of this paper was supported by grants from the Lilly Endowment and the Spencer Foundation.

> wiles of our sex. Never let anyone guess you have a mind of your own." And she made as if to guide my pen. . . . I turned upon her and caught her at the throat. I did my best to kill her. I acted in self defense. Had I not killed her, she would have killed me. She would have plucked the heart out of my writing. (pp. 58-59)

Such an Angel hovered over my initial forays into clinical psychology and my training as a psychotherapist. After reading Virginia Woolf, I named her "the Angel in the Consulting Room." She was so perceptive; she picked up my love of words, my love affair with language, and interfered with my writing too. She would say, "My dear, I am so pleased that you are writing. But perhaps you might begin to modulate your voice a little." But this was after I'd known her for some time.

Let me try to tell the story of how she entered my life. At the age of thirteen I woke from the long dream of childhood and was certain that I was a witch. With uncanny accuracy, I saw myself and others in a new way: suddenly, I could look into the life of the dream, the soul, one ear to the underground. I could see in one swift glance what I was not meant to know – for instance, I saw that one of my teachers was jealous and longed for the easy, free conversations I had with another teacher. But when I asked about this directly, she laughed and said, "No, I don't feel jealous. Where did you ever get such an idea?" Her voice, a tense voice edged with too much dismay, carried another message: "Yes, that's how I feel, but I don't want to talk about it." At first I persisted in speaking about what I saw and heard, felt and thought, even in the face of such discouragement. Soon I got the message more directly: "This cannot be true." "You are making this up." "You must be imagining things." In my confusion about what I could and could not say, in my outrage and loneliness, I began to read a new set of books – the clinical literature I found surreptitiously in my neighborhood library. As I started to read therapists' descriptions of their patients, even with the very first phrases, I felt physically uncomfortable. This was a bodily knowledge, a discomfort so insistent that I could not read for long. But I persisted, not knowing what I needed to know. Looking back on those years, I can see that I identified deeply with the patients, wildly hoping for an authentic, and therefore healing, relationship for myself. Yet what I heard in those clinical case studies, what I felt and tasted in my reading, was for the most part the degradation of patients. "Infection in the sentence breeds . . . " (p. 553) writes Emily Dickinson (1890/1960). Many of the volumes on psychotherapy seemed to infect the life of my mind. But I read Hannah Green's *I Never Promised You a Rose Garden* (1964), and heard within that book a different language. I wondered about a different kind of relationship – an honest relationship between a sixteen year old girl, one of the "still fighting sick," (p. 62) and a woman therapist who refused to idealize life or gloss over real anguish. I had long fantasies in Latin class about being in therapy with "Dr. Fried," whom I discovered was really Frieda Fromm Reichman. Eventually, I imagined, she and I would become friends. I sensed that this would not be agreeable to most therapists (see Langs, 1978). Most of the therapists I read wrote in a dense, cryptic language–designed almost purposefully to hide themselves–and I could not imagine having a conversation, a real conversation, with any of them, much less becoming friends. These therapists seemed to possess an effortless authority, a knowledge I could never possess. As if they inhabited some higher realm, they didn't seem to struggle to know what they knew. And when the therapists were women, they seemed a lot like angels to me: possessed of a supernatural knowledge, too good to be true, and invisible to boot. These women, disembodied and remote, had no real influence on my thinking or my fantasy life. Then I turned to the men, who certainly had written more, and who were cited more often.

I read Freud by lining up a series of books on a library table: an English translation of Freud, Webster's English Dictionary, a German dictionary, a Psychiatric dictionary, and my notebook – in which I constructed a glossary of terms and a running log of my questions and observations. After several months I began to know my way around in Freud's cases. I can still see myself pushing back my braids as I hovered over "Dora" (Freud, 1905/1963), then flying to the other end of the table – while all about me old men sat reading books and newspapers calmly. In this way, I began to explore a new landscape: the geography of psychic life. And from there I moved on to others, Jung and Erikson and the ego analysts and object relations theorists. It was the thrill of entering another language, another country, that held me dancing at my library table those Saturday mornings during all the years of my adolescence. In the beginning I wrote down my questions and objections, but they became fewer and fewer. Once I knew the clinical language, I began to forget my questions. And by the time I was sixteen, I was no longer speaking about what I felt and thought, knew and half-guessed. I could not help but notice, however, that I was leading a double life as I tried to hide what I knew at home and in school. I knew the fine layering of feelings (jealousy, anger, love, longing) and their simplification in language; I knew that many women chose to live as if endlessly running from their own truths; I knew how exhausting it was to read the codes of the unspeakable, to filter out the false voices all around me. I sought some confirmation of what I knew in the clinical literature. This sense of being divided – cut off from myself, unable to speak, unable to find confirmation for what I knew – drove me into the world of art and writing, and into the company of artists, who seemed to know much more than the clinicians knew about the details of psychic life. I remained intrigued with clinical texts, with one critical change – by the time I was sixteen, I was altogether sick of identifying with patients. I wanted, more than anything, to be one of the healers, one of the knowledgeable, one of the experts, one of the elect: a psychotherapist. Through this wish, I unwittingly opened a door for the Angel in the Consulting Room to enter, and in she crept, without introducing herself to me very clearly. I did not know how deeply she could interfere with my writing then.

From thirteen to sixteen, I began to draw and to write poetry. I can now see that I was making a desperate attempt to hold onto a sense of a reality, a feeling of being fully alive. So many of my perceptions and feelings did not translate directly into words, and my drawing and writing did not feel entirely satisfying to me. I found the English language itself constraining, so I created another language. I made up my own alphabet, then began with the words, word-thoughts encoded in clustered lines that looked something like Chinese characters. For each word, I created a metaphoric description, a short poem. For instance, I created a character for the word "fear-hope" (the word could also be spelled out in my own alphabet). This word was spoken as "lei-noch." It translates: "Fear-hope, beware the hope of love, fear hope that opens up in the all-colored paper night." This word, like many others, carried both a feeling and an injunction. The "grammar" used to put this word and other words into sentences was associative, not linear. In other words, the logic was psychological. These words, unlike English words, actually meant different things in their different combinations.

During my adolescence then, I actually had two "new" languages – a growing clinical language pencilled on the pages of school notebooks, and my own language that no one could read or decipher. The language I'd created myself held everything that I thought of as unspeakable and vulnerable: my unanswered questions, my real thoughts and deepest longings. I treasured it and felt the power of this language as healing. But I also felt deeply ashamed of what I'd created and did not share it with anyone. This move to take my voice out of the world allowed me to preserve an authentic writing voice, but at a tremendous cost – I began to believe that what I knew could not thrive in the open air of relationships (see also Brown, in press; Brown and Gilligan, 1990; Gilligan, 1990; Rogers, 1990b). My language proved to be one of the strongest holds of resistance against the Angel in the Consulting Room. I think now that mastering the language of clinical practice threatened to undermine that resistance and prepared the way for a sense of shame, for learning to hate and keep secret what I felt was most truthful in myself. And once I learned that language, I began to be haunted by Woolf's Angel in the House. In her presence, I would try to write "Psychology," glossing over the meanings of the words, taking in the voices of therapists as if they were my own. Then I could feel helpful and knowledgeable and even pure. I wanted to be free of all that tormented and haunted me, so I sided with the Angel, who assured me that with enough time and sacrifice, therapy and training, I too could become a therapist.

This was an uneasy alliance. At times, when I was in the presence of a strong, honest and playful woman (an irregular occurrence in my adolescence), the Angel would seemingly go off on vacation. Then I would read another "case history" and feel with an unsettling clarity my healthy suspicion of the remote therapist who wrote in such a bizarre language, who seemed so inhumanly clean.

When I began my clinical training, the Angel started following me everywhere, into my classes and into my first "practicum." I will introduce her more fully, as I came to know her during those first years of my graduate work, and as I know her now. She resembles Woolf's Angel in her sympathy, unselfishness, loyalty, and purity. She interferes with my writing, as she did with Woolf's. She muffles my voice, erases my thought half finished, and scrambles my arguments into contradictions. She anticipates the responses of others, inserts doubts into plain words, and requires me to protect the feelings of others by silencing myself. She tells me what I write is preposterous and outrageous on the one hand, and on the other that my observations and questions are dull – therefore I should not speak them aloud and embarrass myself publicly.

I do enthusiastic battle with her as I write. And not only would I throw an inkpot at her, but also chairs, glasses of water, and my computer keyboard, an object Woolf didn't have at her disposal. She delights in criticizing what I'm writing now and in making dire predictions about its fate in the world. She whispers to me that what I have written is unclear and incomplete, and warns me that others will dismiss me as "naive" or judge me as "disturbed." When I persist in writing, she sends me nightmares: I speak and the words are gibberish in my mouth; I speak while being strangled, being burned, while falling. Then, waking from such nightmares, when I am really prepared to fight with the Angel, she does not want to "argue." She is hurt and offended, elusive and unreachable. In the end, I am almost always the one who seeks her out – to ask forgiveness, do favors, inquire about her thoughts, feelings, her wishes, her needs – and to watch for some small sign that she still loves me in her own tormented and tormenting way. I do not know if it is worse when she forgives me, or when she does not. It is a false love she offers, I know, but her hand as it brushes the rim of my collar is soft and warm, and perhaps, I think, this is better than nothing. So I have settled for this and have not succeeded in killing her off, though sometimes she leaves me to my solitude for a few hours. Then I write, as if there will never be time enough, as if time is endless, in my own clear voice. Then, sometimes briefly, I can imagine my words going out into the world, their clear tones touching everything lightly, their echoes coming back into the room where I sit writing, and go on writing.

TWO PLAYING: JAMIE AND ANNIE

I look up from my computer keyboard. Sunlight glances off the windowpane, and beyond the glass, melting snow falls from the eaves of the house. I drift into another time. It is twilight and I am lying on my back in the snow in front of the St. Louis State Hospital laughing, making snow angels with Jamie, a thirteen year old girl. Snow falls upward and dances above us before it falls down upon us. We move our arms in great swishing motions to form the wings, reach up above our heads to draw our halos in the snow, then lie still, feeling the cold coming through our coats. "We had better go back," I say aloud. Jamie climbs out of her angel imprint, scattering snow about. She reaches down for my hands and helps pull me to my feet. We walk side by side toward the lights. It is twilight and the old brick buildings, now lit up, cast shadows and little dabs of yellow on the new snow. Jamie walks along in silence. Before we are swallowed up in the entrance, she turns suddenly. "You will never really leave me, will you?" she asks, her voice low. I look at her, this child, her dark hair blowing out in the wind, her dark eyes deeper than puddles after a rain. In my silence, she looks down at her fingers. Her red fingers stick out from the unravelled ends of her dirty gray gloves. It is hard to know what to say. I know what I "should" say. It takes only moments, when time holds still like this, for the sky to darken, going from lilac to violet to blackness. The trees behind us are blurred in darkness already and the snow has already begun to erase our snow angels. I put my arm around Jamie's shoulder. "No, I don't think I will ever have to do that," I tell her – more wish than fact – but it comforts us momentarily.

I was in my early twenties then, working in my first clinical "practicum" on an adolescent ward of a large State Hospital. I saw some of the children individually, but I also just "hung around," as I was doing that evening with Jamie. Often I carried with me boxes of art supplies. Jamie was not on my official roster of patients. She was one of the kids with whom I developed a close relationship, however. A skinny girl with dark uncombed hair, she did not speak to me at first. She sat alone, drawing from a distance by the radiator in the corner of the "dayroom." From time to time, I felt her studying me, but whenever I looked at her, she was bent over a sketch pad. Folded up drawings began to appear near my boxes, with no signature. The drawings were stunning in their detail, and also unsettling – the face of a young girl in black and white with pieces of rice paper glued over the eyes and mouth; a drawing of flowers, each one exquisite, each one torn with a jagged edge of red; and then a series: charcoal drawings of knives, each one intricately wrought. Jamie came and went for most of the autumn while I piled up her drawings, and hid them – for her, for myself. I wondered sometimes if I should speak to someone about the drawings, about Jamie herself, but I did not.

One evening, when she sat hunched over a sketch pad, Jamie rolled up one of her sleeves and began to cut her inner arm with a piece of glass – without expression, apparently without pain. When I realized what she was doing, I wrestled the glass from her hand and threw it across the room. Jamie began to scream, struggling against me to go and recover the glass. Footsteps in the hall – a nurse and two male attendants ready to swarm upon us with needles – "No," I said, "We're doing just fine," my heart pounding. They hesitated, then left us. I dragged Jamie, tense and struggling, to an old green stuffed chair. I pulled her onto my lap, and still she struggled. But suddenly, she went limp and began to cry convulsively, burying her face in my shoulder. I held her for a long time that night, rocking her.

I began to "see" Jamie individually after that, never officially, but very regularly. We would sit outside in the cold courtyard on a green wooden bench, drinking hot cocoa, and in warmer weather, grape soda. We sat together, our bodies close, touching, side by side, in a silence too full for words. And then the stories of her abuse came pouring out. Jamie had been beaten and sexually molested by her step-father since she was six, when he came to live with her family. She did not feel that her mother could believe her or would be able to protect her, and she did not consider telling anyone outside the family. When the haunting shame of her complicity (her simple child's desire for warmth and affection from her step-father) came into her stories, Jamie said, "You will hate me, now." "No," I told her, "Not hate, more like love, Jamie, and your feelings, I have felt those feelings too. Our lives are not so different really." I felt her fingers come into my hand then. I never spoke about this, this conversation, this joining, this love – with my clinical supervisor, or with any of my student colleagues. I sensed that I would endanger my love for this girl, my capacity to be with her, if I were to speak about it.

But I was also afraid for Jamie in that hospital – a place ruled by drugs, behavior modification charts, and periodic evaluations: tests, followed by case conferences. So I began to coach her to cheat on the tests and to disguise what she knew and what she felt – to go underground in order to protect herself and then to get out. But she was terrified that I wanted to "get rid" of her. We fought about this. And I felt like a fraud, fighting to get her out of the hospital, a dangerous place to be sure; but with no assurance of continuing our relationship, I was also sending her into unspeakable danger within. I sensed this, but could not name it, and in my quandary I went to talk to my supervisor about Jamie.

Ruth was a deeply respected child psychologist who had worked with adolescents for over fifteen years. She was fond of me in a rather remote way, but I knew how to read the signs of her affection. She was a tall woman with greying dark hair and piercing blue eyes and often I caught her studying me when I sat in case conferences. She was empathic, sympathetic to my dilemma, but she told me what I feared she would say: "You have known Jamie only six months. She is just thirteen; she will forget all about you." I argued with this, trying to describe how Jamie and I had formed a relationship over a period of months, how deeply she trusted me. "You are very good with these children, Annie. Someday you will even be a gifted therapist, I think. But, you are not her official therapist now. You are not her mother. Under these circumstances, you cannot be her friend." "Why can't I be her friend?" I wanted to know. "Because that's not what she needs," Ruth said. What did Jamie need, I wondered, floundering for my own knowledge. I began again. I told Ruth that the relationship I had with Jamie had gone way beyond friendship; I believed it had been healing for her. Ruth smiled at me, a patient smile, as if she expected this. I must have seemed very young to her then. I was very close to tears. Her next statement undid my knowledge of my relationship with Jamie: "Even if you had been Jamie's therapist, you have violated the boundaries of a therapeutic relationship and you have confused her. It would not be in her best interest for you to continue to see her." Her voice was sympathetic, not at all unkind, but her words stung me. These words did not fit my experience, yet I was new to clinical work, and I believed her in those crucial moments. She seemed to possess an effortless authority. She seemed so knowledgeable, so pure in her intentions. By contrast, I felt naive and young, contrary and selfish in my affection for Jamie.

I did not ever visit with Jamie after she left the hospital, an arbitrary decision made just a few days later. In the end, this decision was not made in light of any "progress" she'd made. I was not even there on the day she was "released."

Ruth, my first supervisor, resembled Woolf's Angel in the House uncannily. Like Woolf's Angel, Ruth was sympathetic and kind, unselfish and pure. And when I came to ask her for help with my dilemma, she transformed herself into the modern day version of Woolf's Angel, the figure I call the Angel in the Consulting Room. This Angel, like Woolf's Angel, makes it next to impossible for girls and women to feel and speak their own truths. Why is this so, given the Angel's intention to be genuinely helpful?

Long ago the Angel in the Consulting Room gave up her voice and her mind, so long ago that she does not recognize her loss or remember herself any differently. Empathic, charming, sympathetic and patient, the Angel in the Consulting Room aligns herself with a practice of psychotherapy that deeply undermines girls' and women's knowledge of relationships. Through her empathy and sympathy, she calls forth the deepest wishes and most vital truths in her patients. Then she steps back, removes herself (perhaps hidden even from herself), and encourages her patients to give up or mourn what they wanted, to let go of the wish for a real and enduring relationship. In this way the Angel in the Consulting Room exemplifies the loss she herself has suffered and passes this loss on to another generation of girls. Intending to be helpful, the Angel continues a political and psychological order in which girls and women are glorified as maternal, but remain essentially unmothered within patriarchal cultures (Chesler, 1972). As a girl growing up, I could not fail to discern that many of the girls I knew somehow managed to cut off their love for their mothers during adolescence, to call this love "dependent" or "immature," and to give up even the wish for a real relationship with an adult woman (see also Brown, in press; Gilligan, 1990; Kincaid, 1983; Rogers, 1990b). This was a loss I fought against with all my being – with my own mother and with other women. Yet what I was learning in my early twenties was that "good therapy" depended upon the therapist putting into practice the unspoken cultural injunction that adolescent girls must give up a wish for a real and enduring relationship with women. This left me with a sense of bitterness and impasse about practicing therapy – a growing sense that girls who could still fight for an honest relationship could not win this fight as patients. In the context of therapy, the very frame of the relationship, the rules or "boundaries" of the practice itself, could be used to defeat girls in their struggle. But this clarity came much later.

In my early twenties I was open to Ruth's words and vulnerable to her suggestions. Ruth, the Angel in the Consulting Room, a therapist I liked and respected, entered the house of my shame, gave me the "password" of her clinical knowledge, and utterly destroyed my capacity to love the child Jamie.

But Jamie comes back to me as I sit looking out on the melting snow. Jamie comes back, carrying her silence, her anger, her love – giving me back my earlier courage with her, my love and the betrayal of that love, and my authentic writing voice.

We were two playing, Jamie and I. I had not learned how to remove myself from her, how to be a "container" (Levenson, 1972) of her experience (somehow miraculously separate from mine), or how to be a "love object" to be "found" (Freud, 1916/1958) by her (rather than a young woman who simply loved her). I was familiar enough with these concepts, but did not know clearly how to implement them, so they did not affect my practice. Therefore, I could play with Jamie, bringing myself fully to her. But the language and practice of therapy that I was learning was utterly at odds with this way of playing.

I wish that I knew what I know now – that there are at least two different stories about what was happening in my relationship with Jamie. I wish that I could have listened to both stories, endured the dizzying doubleness of hearing the contradictions, and trusted the authority of my own knowledge.

The first story is familiar to anyone who has learned about how to make use of the "transference" in therapeutic work. Within this story, my wish to continue to see Jamie outside of the hospital would be seen as an "inappropriate" desire on my part, a wish that could be used as grist for the mill of exploring my own problem with "unclear boundaries" in relationships - in my own therapy, or even in a particular kind of supervision. Jamie's gift of her art work and the way that she cut her arm in my presence could be understood as "manipulative" ways that Jamie invited me or "seduced" me to respond to her "inappropriately." In this story of relationships, if I were her therapist, I would explore her disappointment with her own mother, not with me personally. Over time, her disappointment could be analyzed, internalized, and "worked through." In this story, my readiness to hold her, a thirteen year old girl coming into her own sexuality and sexual desire, would also be viewed as "inappropriate," something to be explored as part of my "countertransference" with a supervisor or perhaps in my own therapy. Over time, I would learn through this story of relationships that Jamie had to understand her wishes differently – she had to learn to "contain" them and not to "act them out." And I would learn (like any "good therapist") to empathize with girls in Jamie's position, but not to respond so spontaneously, so honestly and playfully, and certainly not to be so easily "seduced" into an "inappropriate relationship."

But there is another story here, another rendering of this relationship, one that is at once familiar to us as women, and also unfamiliar as clinicians, because it runs counter to clinical language and practice. Perhaps Jamie's wish for a real and enduring relationship with me is worth trusting. Through this wish she invites me into a vital drama, a drama in which two are playing and both persons playing are really vulnerable to one another. In this story both the patient and the therapist are capable of accurately knowing and healing one another (also see Heimann, 1950; Searles, 1979). In this story, when a therapist asks a girl to give up her wish for a real and enduring relationship, this request is a sign of the therapist's own loss and a betrayal of her patient's trust. For if her patient gives up this vital wish she must also give up the promise of being able to love deeply and authentically. In this story, Jamie's desire is essentially a healthy desire. If this is the case, Jamie must then find someone who can support her wish – a therapist who can resist the language of the traditional story in order to explore carefully what it might mean to take her wish seriously. In this story, girls' and women's responses to one another – the powerful unconscious interplay Freud (1912/1958) labelled "transference" and "countertransference" (after all, what love does not transfer or spill over from one relationship to the next?) – may be, but are not necessarily distortions. The fine interplay of responses that makes psychotherapy so deeply enchanting and powerful, so difficult for both therapist and patient at times, is a source of healing for both.

How do I know this story? How do I claim any authority whatsoever for this version of a healing relationship? Through the authority of my own experience with Jamie I know this story. It was Jamie, after all, "one of the still fighting sick," who watched me and waited for some sign (perhaps it was my collecting and saving her drawings) that it might be worth her trouble to test my strength as a fighter. If I listen for her unspoken questions, a knowledge expressed through her self mutilation because it cannot be spoken directly, I hear her asking me, an adult woman: Will you fight against my destruction? Will you fight for a real relationship with me? Will you fight with your whole being for this? Jamie is very astute about finding a real relationship at thirteen, as are other girls who are not in psychiatric hospitals but who resist false relationships (see Brown and Gilligan, 1990; Rogers, 1990b). Jamie is in fact so psychologically and physically "literate" in reading my responses to her that she knows exactly how to play out this vital drama – and, not unlike a very fine actor, she draws me immediately into a powerful scene, wounding herself with the glass. She comes alive with me only after we have struggled physically. And she speaks with me about her abuse only after we have waited for her words, waited in a silence too full for words, sitting side by side on a green bench. I think none of this would have been possible for Jamie if she had not discovered first that I would fight for her with all my strength, not with needles. But I did not know, as I sat rocking her that night, that she could and would also push me into the most critical questions about my training as a psychotherapist.

Jamie, like other adolescent girls who come into therapy still vital and alive, carries a question, a problem as yet unsolved in any systematic practice of psychotherapy: If the survival of girls' knowledge of real relationships and the survival of their courage depends upon girls' relationships with women, how can girls heal women therapists so that women may in turn heal girls?

A SKETCH OF THE PAST: RESISTANCE TO CLINICAL TRAINING

This question has haunted me for the past eight years of my life. What follows is a quick sketch of the recent past, a gesture drawing of associations and feelings, a vanishing-into-metaphors sort of thinking, the sky-writing of my ongoing dilemma with clinical training and practice.

I forgot the story of my experience with Jamie until recently, though the notes in my journals left a clear trace of our relationship, including verbatim conversations. Jamie abandoned and then forgotten. Amnesia. The snow angels erased. Falling snow that went on falling, burying love. And, like any loved but neglected ghost, Jamie haunted me. I turned away from her and started graduate studies in English Literature.

I was hungry for words, for novels and poetry, for the great comfort of the Oxford English Dictionary in bed at night. Trying to free up words again, to reclaim the richness of words, old words, I rediscovered Chaucer and the Wife of Bath's Tale (1963). Reading her tale as a struggle to know what she knew, to resist the authorities of her day and to claim her own full authority, I thought I'd found a character as different from Woolf's Angel and the Angel in the Consulting Room as could be found anywhere. In her company, I began to write poetry again. But I could not stop thinking about clinical practice.

When I switched programs and took up clinical training in Psychology again, one year later, turning away from writing, poetry trickled down into a dry stream bed. Despite this loss, I was not terribly unhappy. I was fascinated by the life of the mind, as I had been at thirteen, intrigued by learning the detailed process of psychotherapeutic work. But I doubled as a resistant ghost writer. The ghost writer wrote in light pencil all the things I knew I was not supposed to think and feel, and her irreverent questions filled the margins of my books and notebooks. "Why would generations of therapists, men and women alike, adopt a language of distance and condescension, a tone of false authority, and then absent themselves almost entirely from their own writing?" she wrote. On another page, she scribbled, "Who or what are they protecting?" And everywhere I turned – in my own therapy with a feminist therapist, in my classes, and in my internships – I sensed a sham of a healing relationship, and felt an almost irrepressible impulse to disrupt and somehow expose this sham of love. What words could I use to speak about love when I was learning to sell myself as a "love object" in psychotherapy? What about the patients who, like Jamie, would wish for real love? Would girls and women then pay me as a therapist for the fulfillment of a sham of love and learn to call it love? It seemed to me that this was the usual practice. No one spoke about this. No one even had these questions. The Angel in the Consulting Room lived everywhere around me, a woman welcome in this culture, a woman welcome in the professional world I was entering.

I tried to join this professional world, the world of clinical practice. And I found that I could work with some feeling of integrity only with adult schizophrenics or very disturbed children because their disturbances made them so startlingly honest. I found a child analyst to work with, a woman who had great confidence in me and who did not argue with my interpretations or my way of playing with my young patients. I talked quite openly with her about what I said and did. But my experiences in supervision had shaken my faith in truth-telling, and I told her remarkably little about my life. And of course, I did not tell her about Jamie or Ruth because I had forgotten them. Most critically, I could not raise with her my most unsettling questions about clinical practice.

I finished my internship and my degree and then, unlike the other students in my program, I stopped practicing altogether.

A FEMINIST POETICS OF PSYCHOTHERAPY

I sit at my computer, thinking about why I stopped practicing and looking out on the dingy snow, bright in the mid-afternoon light. I catch children's voices as they cross the street here, going home from school. I imagine Jamie among them. It is Jamie herself whom I recognize. She appears unchanged – still thirteen with dark hair and eyes, those eyes that see so much, so quickly, and though I am afraid, I am drawn to her as I was years ago.

How was it possible for me to join with the Angel in the Consulting Room and to forget my love for Jamie? What did I know (that I could not let myself know) that Ruth perhaps did not know? With this question, the Angel enters the room where I sit writing. The shadow of her wings falls on my hands. "This question is not worth your trouble," she says. "First of all, you are assuming that you knew something Ruth did not, and there you were, a young woman, naive and inexperienced as a clinician. Please don't write this way about something that you know so little about." She puts her hands on my shoulders. "I am only saying this to protect you," she adds. Her presence, her hands, her voice in my ears, throws me off center, off voice. How badly I want to fight with her about this! But I know that I could be damaged fighting with her. If I were to touch the place where she has been wounded as a woman in this culture, in all likelihood she would react defensively, and then she could so easily use the language and structure of psychotherapy to protect herself. So, if I were to really resist her, to fight for a real relationship with her, I might damage myself deeply. Fear lights the edges of the room.

Jamie was able to fight with me, she fought with me quite consistently about leaving, and she came very close to healing me: "You are just trying to get rid of me," she would begin. "You don't really love me anymore." I remember her standing by a radiator in the back hallway late one afternoon during such an argument, her back turned toward me. I tried to reassure her that I did not want to get rid of her at all, and that I loved her as much as ever. I reached out to touch her shoulder, but she pulled away from my touch, would not even meet my eyes that day. I remember how petulant she seemed to me, how helpless and furious with her I felt that day. Now, I stand in wonder of her courage. She did not fudge the truth about her fear of my betrayal, not one bit. And her fear was realistic. Her accusation that I was trying to "get rid" of her touched a sore spot, a place where I was wounded (after all, I could listen to Ruth, the Angel in the Consulting Room, and take her more seriously than Jamie herself). I drew back from this pain, unable to name it.

"My dear, be careful now," the Angel interjects.

What is this white wall of terror? Why in the course of writing this paper does my skin burn? What is it that I am so terrified to know? What is the parallel process between what girls like Jamie experience with women in therapy and what I have experienced in the clinical world myself? Why did I stop practicing?

I can't write now where can I go now my skin burns can't write like this voices quiet not knowing please let my tongue come unglued let the words come what would be the worst love that isn't love, no, not again, no, never, but now running from all this fear I hate her I love her running into burning fear not angels not women where are the letters the words my hands won't work burning not to know to know not to speak go through the fire burned in this fire what is really happening to me what is love stop this please all this running into memories of what she can she can't there not there maddening how can women heal girls when girls can't even say can't even feel or speak what they know in therapy?

"Of course girls can speak about what they know in therapy," the Angel says gently. "*I* would really work hard to hear and accept whatever you said, to be with you, to help you," she goes on. Her voice is soft and low. How can I get angry with someone so sympathetic and helpful? She touches my longing for a mother, or at least for the shadow of a lost mother. I could settle for this – the crumbs of her help – and try to believe her words. If I do not kill her, she will kill me. She will insert doubts into everything that I've written in this paper. And then? I would feel mad. I would be so out of touch with the reality of my own experience, and so dissociated from my own voice and knowledge, as to be mad.

Fighting with the Angel is the unimaginable response that I know could save us. And for all my complaints about her, I do love her. Could I engage her in a real fight? Could I touch her wound, open it, and let her in turn heal me? And if I could do this, would it make any difference to other women and girls? What would my friend Virginia Woolf do?

Woolf was compelled to fight and kill the Angel in the House in order to write (for writing truthfully is utterly at odds with the Angel's sensibilities). So girls, particularly adolescent girls who are resisters, may be compelled to fight the Angel in the Consulting Room. Better that girls should kill the Angel in their women therapists than kill themselves or give up the hope for a real relationship altogether. The capacity to fight the Angel on the part of a single girl (perhaps a girl like Jamie), may then stir in a woman (as it has in me) memories of herself (also see Gilligan, 1990, p. 531). She may then recall herself as a girl who loved freely and fiercely. She may then remember a time before the loss of voice and the pervasive sense of abandonment that adolescent girls experience so commonly in this culture (Brown, in press; Gilligan 1990; Rogers, 1990b). She may then begin to wonder if her own loss and the rage that trailed in its wake was not altogether necessary. Then such a woman may be able to join the girl who is her patient in fighting and in killing the Angel who interferes with their work together and who undermines their love and knowledge.

In fighting with their therapists, girls may be able to disrupt radically an inauthentic relationship and to heal their women therapists, so that women may in turn heal girls. This resistance on the part of girls, however, depends upon their potential to be taken seriously in such a struggle. In order for me to join even a single girl in her resistance (also see Gilligan, 1990), I discovered that I had to write against the Angel in the Consulting Room, write my way into a different discourse – a feminist poetics of psychotherapy. I have had to re-enter (stepping into a clear bath) a lucid, poetic language, a language that floods me with memories of myself as a girl and spills over into poetry. My words enter a sea of relationships with women who grew up and struggled for their own love and knowledge one generation ahead of me. I wrote the following poem about what I learned in one of these relationships:

And she came to tell me, her eyes lit up,
about "No!" and "Not me!" –laughing
in a mirror game. Turning in her long blue dress
and petticoat, she whispers a tacit promise –
and is this love?
And she came to tell me about one button
missing from her blue sweater
that sits by the tea cup on the sink
waiting to be sewn back on. Things
pop up, pop open, pop off: buttons and words,
milkweed pods and love . . . Sometimes
my mind flies with hers in silence,
and sometimes need
comes creeping back downstairs,
surprising me – hello cat.
And she came to tell me how that morning
entering her clothes
she thought of taking them off again
and how she went bare breasted, bare backed
out into the rose garden and sat down
in a little pool there.
And she came to tell me that under
three layers of darkness was a fish –
and then how she couldn't get warm,
couldn't get warm – false voices
all around her – and her grandfather
gone. And she came to tell me, at night
you sleep as if by yourself,
but with all those characters in dreams
water falling in great waves and horses running,
the ground dances and embraces you
and you are never, never quite
entirely alone.

Birthday Gift (Rogers, 1990a)

The recovery of this knowledge of relationships among women of different generations is critical to discovering a different practice of healing for girls and women.

In my own tentative and raw new practice with girls, my resistance to the language and rules of traditional psychotherapy, the very way that I learn a different practice, deeply depends upon the resistance of girls. I have begun a practice with a single girl, a girl who came to me just as she turned thirteen – depressed, frightened, struggling to know what she knew – in school, and in her family. Unlike Jamie, Karen was not a fighter from the beginning. Although she has learned to fight within her family and to trust her own knowledge to some degree, she has not yet brought herself as a resister to me. This is a signal that something is amiss in my practice. I am waiting for her to fight with me, to resist what is still problematic in my practice. When that time comes, I wonder if I will be able to kill the Angel in the Consulting Room (you have noticed perhaps that I have not done this), and then to travel with her into a real and enduring relationship that heals both of us.

REFERENCES

Brown, L. (in press). A problem of vision: The development of relational voice in girls ages 7 to 16. *Women's Studies Quarterly.*

Brown, L., & Gilligan, C. (1990). The psychology of women and the development of girls. Manuscript submitted for publication.

Chaucer, G. (1963). The wife of bath's tale. In A. Baugh (Ed.), *Chaucer's major poetry* (pp. 382-402). Engelwood Cliffs, NJ: Prentice-Hall, Inc.

Chesler, P. (1972). *Women and madness.* New York: Avon Books.

Dickinson, E. (1960). *The complete poems of Emily Dickinson.* Boston: Little, Brown and Company. (Original work published in 1890).

Freud, S. (1963). Dora: *An analysis of a case of hysteria.* New York: Macmillan. (Original work published in 1905).

Freud, S. (1958). The dynamics of transference. *Standard edition, 12* (pp. 99-108). London: Hogarth Press. (Original work published in 1912).

Freud, S. (1958). *Introductory lectures on psychoanalysis.* London: Hogarth Press. (Original work published in 1916).

Gilligan, C. (1990). Joining the resistance: Psychology, politics, girls and women. *Michigan Quarterly Review, 29*(4), 501-536.

Green, H. (1964). *I never promised you a rose garden.* New York: The New American Library, Inc.

Heimann, P. (1950). On countertransference. *International Journal of Psycho-analysis, 31*, 81-84.
Kincaid, J. (1983). *Annie John.* New York: Farrar, Straus and Giroux.
Langs, R. (1978). *Technique in transition.* New York: Jason Aronson, Inc.
Levenson, E. (1972). *The fallacy of understanding.* New York: Basic Books.
Rogers, A. (1990a). Birthday gift. Unpublished poem.
Rogers, A. (1990b). The development of courage in girls and women. Unpublished manuscript, Harvard University, Project on the Psychology of Women and the Development of Girls, Cambridge, MA.
Searles, H. (1979). *Countertransference.* New York: International Universities Press.
Woolf, V. (1944). *A Haunted House and Other Stories.* New York: Harcourt, Brace and World. (Original work published in 1921).

Adolescent Girls, Women and Sexuality: Discerning Dilemmas of Desire

Deborah L. Tolman

I. FEMALE ADOLESCENT SEXUAL DESIRE: A CONUNDRUM

In her 1987 paper "Clarity in Connection: Empathic Knowing, Desire and Sexuality," Judith Jordan has taken the lead in grappling with some troubling questions about female sexuality. She has engaged in a risky and admirable struggle to explain her own and other clinicians' pervasive observation that women have trouble knowing their own sexual desire. In this paper, she suggests that women's lack of clarity about their own desire may be rooted in a developmental difference between girls and boys that occurs in adolescence. She outlines two developmental paths in adolescence, the emergence in boys of "sexual entitlement" and in girls of "sexual accommodation" which leads to a lack of clarity for females about their own desire. Jordan says that she has not heard her women patients speak about an "explosion of sexual impulses in adolescence" (p. 14). In her view, the central dynamic of female sexuality is the relational context; in sexual terms, the "primary needs" of females are "the need not to be used, and to be empathically validated and 'emotionally held'" (p. 15). She posits an alternative

---

Deborah L. Tolman is Assistant Project Director of the research study "Understanding Adolescents At-Risk" and is a member of the Harvard Project on the Psychology of Women and the Development of Girls. Her current research is a qualitative study of adolescent girls' experiences of sexual desire. She is also engaged in training in feminist psychotherapy. Preparation of this paper was supported in part by the Boston Foundation.

conception of desire that highlights the experience of women, a relational model of desire, "contextual desire," which is the "desire for the experience of joining toward and joining in something that thereby becomes greater than the separate selves" (p. 11) and is "informed by empathic knowing of the other" (p. 18). Jordan suggests that women's lack of clarity about their own desire emerges out of the failure of a woman's male sexual partner to be empathically aware of her desire as an aspect of his own desire; this absence of empathy thus makes it difficult for a woman to have clarity about her own desire.

I am interested specifically in the tension which runs through this paper. Jordan makes the observation that the sexual activity in which adolescent girls and women engage is physically exciting to them: "I am not suggesting that girls don't become powerfully aroused in the early adolescent explorations of kissing and fondling . . . and women are clearly capable of powerful, intense orgasms" (p. 16). Jordan has stated her knowledge that adolescent girls can and do experience intense embodied sexual desire, yet she leaves out this bodily fact in how she speaks about the adolescent girl as centrally "interested in closeness, tenderness, being loved" (p. 16) when it comes to sex. Despite Jordan's knowledge that sexual desire, excitement and pleasure occur in female bodies, embodied sexual hunger is curiously missing as a fundamental aspect of female sexuality in the relational model she is exploring. An ambivalence seems to run through this paper, as Jordan speaks about the importance of "attunement to our bodies" (p. 17) yet emphasizes only the relational aspects of female sexual experience, focusing on women's lack of clarity about sexual desire.

Jordan concludes that little is known about the development of female sexuality and that "the picture of adolescent sexuality is still heavily colored by the male experience" (p. 16). But she does have some knowledge about adolescent female sexual desire – that girls can "become powerfully aroused." By discounting her own knowledge of embodied female sexual feelings, she overlooks the tension between what she knows and what is missing in what she hears her clients say about their adolescent experience. Jordan honors her clients' experiences and tries to understand what they have told her through a relational model of female sexuality. But when she leaves aside their bodies in framing and understanding their experience as essentially relational, she loses what might be an important question: If I know that adolescent girls can experience sexual excitement in their bodies, why don't I hear about embodied sexual desire when adolescent girls talk of their sexual experience or in women's recollections of their adolescent sexual experience? I am struck that Jordan knows that adolescent girls have embodied sexual feelings and yet she does not wonder about the absence of physical sexual desire in what women and adolescent girls say about their adolescent sexual experience.

II. THE MISSING DISCOURSE OF DESIRE: A DILEMMA FOR ADOLESCENT GIRLS

Jordan's willingness to think out loud about the conundrum of sexual desire in female adolescence is, as Irene Stiver observes in the discussion summary of the paper, deserving of congratulations. She is, in fact, speaking into a deafening silence within the psychological literature. Outside of the domain of psychology, however, feminist writers have been naming and exploring the absence of female sexual desire in Western patriarchal culture's conceptions of female sexuality for the past fifteen years (i.e., Hite, 1976; Snitow, Stansell and Thompson, 1983; Vance, 1984). Having revealed the silencing, denigration and obscuring of female sexual desire that androcentric notions of female sexuality served, feminists are now exploring what female sexual desire is. A number of feminist scholars have built on Foucault's (1978) analysis that discourse about sexuality – the terms, tenor and tone in which sexuality is talked about – shapes sexual experience and that discourse is controlled and deployed by those in power (Duggan, 1990; Rubin, 1984; Snitow, Stansell and Thompson, 1983; Vance, 1984); a number of French feminists are engaged in creating a way of speaking about female sexual desire, ecriture feminine – writing the body – that they suggest does not exist in "phallocentric" language (Cixous, 1981; Irigaray, 1981, 1985; see also Dallery, 1989). These writers emphasize that what we do and do not say, what we do and do not hear, about sexual desire is a critical shaping force of our capacity to acknowledge, understand and respond to the feelings in our bodies. It is interesting to note that few feminist scholars consider specifically the experience of adolescent girls in their analyses of female sexual desire (Tolman, 1990). Jordan senses that the lack of clarity about desire she hears from women may have something to do with the development of sexuality in adolescence. The silence about adolescent girls' sexual desire has only recently been acknowledged and broken.

In her 1988 article "Sexuality, Schooling, and Adolescent Females: The Missing Discourse of Desire," feminist psychologist Michelle Fine reports her observation that a discourse of desire is missing from the ways in which adolescent female sexuality is conceived of and discussed by teachers and administrators in schools. Girls' sexuality was a topic of discussion but only spoken about in the condoned sexuality discourses, each of which discourages girls' sexual exploration: the discourse of victimization, that girls are taken advantage of by boys; the discourse of disease, that girls need to avoid being infected by sexually transmitted diseases and AIDS; and the discourse of morality, that girls need to behave in a moral fashion that does not include sexual activity. I have searched the literature on adolescent sexuality and female development for theoretical or empirical work on girls' sexual desire (Tolman, 1990). There has been no research by psychologists on female adolescent sexual desire; the major developmental theories since Freud have not only left out girls' experience (Gilligan, 1977, 1982), they have also muted sexual desire as a central dynamic in adolescent development, moving development out of the body, first into society and then into the mind.[1] Even feminist theories of female development have been silent about adolescent girls' sexual desire (i.e., Chodorow, 1974,1989; Gilligan, 1977, 1982; Miller, 1976, 1984; Surrey, 1984). The glossing over of adolescent girls' sexual desire that Fine encountered in schools and that I discovered in the literature of developmental psychology reflects the missing discourse of adolescent girls' sexual desire in society at large.

From the perspective of feminist analyses of female sexual desire, Michelle Fine began to hear a discourse of adolescent girls' desire in schools when she started to listen to girls themselves; she heard it as "a whisper. . . an interruption of the ongoing conversation" (Fine, 1988, p. 33) articulated by girls themselves. By listening carefully to what girls said in schools when they spoke about their sexuality in bathrooms, classrooms and in conversations with her, Michelle Fine discerned some girls weaving a discourse of desire, a naming of their own embodied longing for sexual pleasure, through the ways in which they talked about their sexual experience. Because this discourse of desire was missing in the condoned discourses of adolescent female sexuality in schools, girls' sexual desire was neither audible nor knowable to most of the adults, however. In Fine's view, the absence of an acknowledgement of girls' embodied sexual feelings is a problem. She suggests that this missing discourse may result in girls' failure to know themselves as the subjects of their own sexuality. If girls could conceive of themselves as sexual subjects, they could then potentially make decisions about their sexual behavior and experience that would be healthy for them.

Coming of age in a culture in which their embodied sexual desire is silenced, obscured and denigrated poses a problem for girls. Adolescent girls get a clear message that they are not supposed to become aroused; they hear what the discourses spoken within dominant culture frame for them as their sexual experience – the discourses of victimization, disease and morality that Fine heard spoken in schools. Yet as Judith Jordan (1987) points out, girls' bodies "become powerfully aroused" (p. 16). The tension that I perceive running through Jordan's paper may in fact be the struggle that adolescent girls themselves are engaged in. If girls know about their sexual desire from their experience of their own bodies but encounter a disembodied way of speaking, hearing, and knowing about their sexuality, then a central dilemma is posed for adolescent girls: In what relationship can an adolescent girl be with her sexual desire, with her own body, with her own experience? How do girls both take in the messages from the culture (Gilligan, 1990; Gilligan, Brown and Rogers, 1990) that encourage them not to know their sexual desire and also stay connected to their own bodily experience?

If I tune my ears to listening for dilemmas which can arise when girls do speak about their own sexual feelings, these feelings that no one names, in what girls say when they speak about their sexuality, I can hear some girls struggling with this problem. Listen to the words of Anne Frank, writing to Kitty, the persona of her diary, about her conundrum:

> Once more there is a question which gives me no peace: 'Is it right? Is it right that I should have yielded so soon, that I am so ardent, just as ardent and eager as Peter himself? May I, a girl, let myself go to this extent?' . . . I am afraid of myself, I am afraid that in my longing I am giving myself too quickly. (cited in Dalsimer, 1986, p. 67)

Anne knows and names the feelings of sexual desire in her body – she is "ardent and eager;" she experiences "longing." But she understands also that she, "a girl," should not "let herself go" and be "giving [her]self too quickly." Coming up against what she has learned is appropriate for a girl in the 1944 culture of Western Europe to feel and to do, Anne ponders "a question which gives [her] no peace." I can hear Anne struggling with the dilemma that emerges, precisely because she is keenly aware of both her own sexual desire and the cultural prohibition against her feeling or responding to her sexual feelings. Carol Gilligan has observed that, elsewhere in her diary, Anne Frank raises questions about how this culture dismisses women, and how women do not fight to be known in ways that reflect the reality of their experience (Gilligan, 1990); Gilligan observes that Anne resists taking in what the culture says about women and female experience when it runs counter to her own experience. Here too, I think Anne has painted a self-portrait of resistance to messages about her sexuality, but the dilemma that results from her resistance is obvious: If she knows that she has sexual feelings and, at the same time, she knows that she is not supposed to feel this way as a girl, how can she both have these feelings and be an acceptable girl?

Now I listen to the words of a 16-year-old girl, speaking fifty years later, in a note written to her psychiatrist. After the sexual revolution and the enormous changes that have taken place in how society responds to female sexuality, this girl is caught in the same dilemma in which Anne found herself, struggling between her experience of sexual desire and knowing that she's "not supposed to get excited:"

> I don't know how to bring up the subject of these feelings I get. Girls aren't supposed to – they're not supposed to get excited . . . It's hard to know what to think about this subject. I wake up, and I've had a dream and I'm all excited because of the dream, I think. So then my body starts moving on me. Do you know what I mean? I'm not sure I do, myself! I'm sorry I can't write better. I mean, express myself. That's the worst part of being a teenager, there's so much going on inside you, but you can't talk to anyone about it, even to your closest friend . . . I'll be thinking about this boy in school, and I get worked up . . . I saw this movie 'Cat on a Hot Tin Roof,' and I thought to myself, that's you, and when will you get off the roof, or when will the roof quiet down? (Coles, 1985, pp. 4-5)

Coles pronounces her "forthright" (p. 5) but does not notice that she is speaking about how she is not supposed to notice sexual feelings in her body or talk about these feelings, *because* she is a girl: "Girls aren't supposed to – they're not supposed to get excited." Confused by the contradiction that her own experience makes visible, she knows that she has these feelings but says she does not know – "Do you know what I mean? I'm not sure I do myself" – and in this way starts to "undo" what she has said about her knowledge of her own sexual excitement and the cultural ban on those feelings. She is articulate and "forthright," yet she says she "can't write" or "express herself." Coles concludes that her struggle is a typical adolescent concern about normality, missing entirely that her conflict is about being a girl who gets sexually excited in the context of a culture that says she is not supposed to feel this way. He does not hear that she is trying to resist messages that run counter to her own bodily feelings.

Both Anne Frank and Coles' patient seem to be in a process of resistance against taking in the message that they do not and cannot have sexual desire. As resisters, these girls are probably more the exception than the rule; because adolescent girls live in a culture which obscures, denigrates, silences and is silent about their desire, I think that most girls can and will speak in the voice of the culture. If no one around them speaks about girls' desire, then girls may have trouble speaking directly themselves. The missing discourse of desire that pervades Western culture then creates a problem both for girls and for therapists, as well as other adult women working with adolescent girls: How can we hear and speak to girls about the feelings they have in their bodies, if we hear and speak in the socially condoned missing discourse of their desire – which girls themselves may have taken in?

III. RESPONSIVE/RESISTING LISTENING: HEARING/EXPLORING GIRLS' MISSING DISCOURSE OF DESIRE

Even when we as women begin to listen to girls with a clear understanding both of their potential to feel sexual desire and the knowledge that this desire is not talked about in dominant Western culture, it can still be hard to hear adolescent girls speak about their desire. While Michelle Fine writes eloquently about girls' discourse of desire, in the few examples of girls speaking about desire that pepper her text, their discourse of desire is difficult to discern. For instance, an example in the article which illustrates girls' discourse of desire is one girl's explanation for not showing up for an interview: "my boyfriend came home from the Navy and I wanted to spend the night with him, we don't get to see each other much" (p. 33). This reference to desire is almost like a code; it is hard to pick up unless one has a key. Another feminist scholar, Sharon Thompson, struggles to hear girls speak about their sexual desire and pleasure in the 400 narratives about sexuality, reproduction and romance she has collected (Thompson, 1984; 1990). She was dismayed to hear most girls speaking not of their own desire but of "the quest romance," not of the sexual excitement and pleasure of initial experiences of intercourse but of pain and boredom. These efforts to hear girls speak about their sexual desire illustrate how hard it may be both for girls to speak and how hard it may be for women to hear a discourse of desire. Girls' discourse of desire may be subtle, encoded in the constricted ways which the culture makes available for them to speak about an unspeakable topic. Or girls may describe their experiences consciously in a missing discourse of desire, knowing full well that they should not name their sexual hunger. Many girls may in fact solve the dilemma of their own sexual desire in the face of a culture that does not acknowledge their bodies by not feeling those feelings. Women who have been sexually abused as adolescents often have difficulty with their sexual desire (Kaplan, 1990; Llera, 1991). They may actually have experienced a doubled disconnection in protecting themselves psychologically by dissociating from their bodies and also in astutely picking up a cultural message not to speak about sexual feelings. Lesbian women, who often report not feeling their sexual feelings until after adolescence (deMonteflores and Schultz, 1978), may come up against a doubled resistance as well; in addition to the missing discourse of desire that all adolescent girls must negotiate, they encounter silence about their sexual desire for women as well.

In order for women to hear girls speak about desire, it may be helpful for women to become responsive/resisting listeners of girls (Brown and Gilligan, 1990). This approach builds on the Reading Guide, a strategy for analyzing girls' narratives about their experience that has been developed by researchers at the Harvard Project for the Psychology of Women and the Development of Girls (see Brown, 1988). It may also be used as a form of clinical listening. Acknowledging that female voice and experience are muffled and silenced in the context of Western culture, this approach enables the reader or listener to "bring to the surface the 'undercurrent' of female voices and visions as it filters through an androcentric culture" (Brown and Gilligan, 1990, p. 4). It is an explicitly psychological method, which encourages the reader to consider the meaning of what is said and what is not said by girls about aspects of their experience that are silenced by the culture and about which girls are encouraged to be silent (Brown et al., in press; Gilligan, Brown and Rogers, 1990; Rogers and Gilligan, 1988). A responsive/resisting listener struggles to connect with what girls do and do not say about their experience by being explicitly grounded in her own experience as female in this culture.

I suggest that we, as therapists and other women working with girls, can use our knowledge that adolescent girls can feel sexual desire, and our awareness of the missing discourse of this desire, in the dominant culture to begin to be responsive/resisting listeners to girls when they speak about their sexuality and sexual experiences, as well as to women recollecting their adolescence. I will present a narrative told by Pamela, a 15-year-old Hispanic girl in a longitudinal study of female development.[2] While this narrative was told to an adult woman in a research interview, this story about girls' sexual experience might also be shared in therapy. Pamela tells this narrative in response to the question: "Can you tell me about a time when you were considering a decision about sex and you had to work something out?"

> I liked this kid in February and . . . I got to know him and I like him but I don't like him as a boyfriend. I like him as a real good friend. Everyone here thinks that we go out, but we are just real good friends . . . For now, I'd say definitely no [to having sex], because I don't want my husband to be like, you are already leftovers you know, so I would want to be, I want to wear white when I get married . . . I know one of my friends, she, I asked her because I knew the kid, . . . I told her, if he asks you are you gonna and she said no, because I used to go out with I don't know who for a year or something and it never came it, well, it did and I said no, I didn't have to do that just to be his girlfriend and all that. So then she's been going out with him for seven months and I know she's already had sex with him about three times or something. So I guess, I guess you can't really say nuthin until the time happens, because she was sure, she was like I'm just going to be like no, Derek, I don't want to do it right now but she said when it came up, it just happened and half of her was like go for it, and the other was like no, you know, your mother. So she said that, she couldn't really say no, it was just was happening and it happened before she even thought about it.

Pamela begins the story by speaking obliquely about how she does not experience desire – "I don't like him as a boyfriend. I like him as a real good friend" translates that she is not sexually interested in him. Pamela explains her very good reasons for "definitely saying no" to sex: She wants to avoid being branded as a girl who desires sex, because she is under enormous pressure, particularly in her context in a traditional Hispanic family (see Espin, 1984), to "wear white when [she] gets married" and to avoid being "leftovers" to her husband. If I listen for how she speaks about herself, I begin to consider how she may be speaking in a missing discourse of desire. I begin to wonder if she may be having physical feelings and how she may be responding to them. Because Pamela speaks clearly in the voice of the culture which will not name her own bodily feelings, it is difficult to know what feelings she may have for the boy who is "just a friend." Is she struggling not to know or feel her own desire? Is she not sexually interested in him, introducing him into the narrative in order to fortify a portrait of herself as a girl who does not feel desire? Is there someone whom she desires who goes unnamed when she speaks in this missing discourse? Or, more simply, does she experience no sexual desire for this particular boy?

Then a tension arises in her story between this description of herself told in missing discourse – "I'd definitely say no . . . I want to wear white" – and her knowledge that girls do experience sexual desire and can end up having sex without intending to. Pamela goes on to tell a story about "Sally," her friend, who, in the face of the dilemma posed by her own desire and her knowledge that she "should" say no, ends up having sex "happen" to her. As responsive/resisting listener, I can pose the question: What is Pamela saying about her knowledge and questions about her own sexual desire by telling this story about another girl? It would be very easy and quite tempting as women in this culture to align with Pamela's circumvented ways of speaking about herself and to remain silent about her missing discourse of desire. It would be so simple to applaud and support her firm claim that she "wants to wear white" when she gets married; after all, this stance would protect her from pregnancy, sexually transmitted diseases and AIDS, and she sounds so clear and confident about this position. So why would I want to identify and explore with Pamela her ways of speaking about sexual feelings and to engage with her in an embodied discourse of desire? While Pamela does not ever name explicitly her own sexual desire or any struggle with it, by telling the story about Sally's sexual experience, she may be cueing me that the picture she has drawn of herself may not be so neat.

As a responsive/resisting listener, I am drawn to how Pamela describes Sally's struggle: "half of her was like go for it and the other was like no, you know, your mother." Pamela lets the listener know that she is aware that girls can have sexual feelings in their bodies – girls may want to go for it" – and that girls know that they are not supposed to respond to these feelings – "no, you know, your mother," which makes Sally's sexual longing problematic. Pamela signals the listener that she may understand that this experience could happen to her as well, despite her clear statement that she "wants to wear white;" she shifts out of the story about Sally, making a more general aside: "I guess you can't really say nuthin until the time happens, because she was sure, she was like 'I'm just going to be like no, Derek, I don't want to do it right now.'" Pamela, too, appears to be sure. But Pamela is under real pressure to take on, live and speak as the image of the bride in white. What purpose does Pamela serve by telling this story about Sally? Does Pamela wonder herself, behind her firm resolve, if she too would want "to go for it?" If Pamela continues to speak in a missing discourse of desire, might she find herself in the same position as Sally? If Pamela can move out of a missing discourse of desire, to know and respond to her own desire, may she be less likely to find sex "just happening" to her and more likely to make responsible choices about what she will and will not do?

In noticing that Pamela is not speaking about her own desire, yet she is letting her listener in on her awareness of other girls' sexual desire, I become curious about Pamela's own sexual feelings and struggles with her body and the messages about it she has taken in. I think the unspoken questions that Pamela seems to be raising in this complicated narrative could go unrecognized quite easily. It would be very easy for me to misalign with the missing discourse she knows so well and, I would imagine, hears from many women in her life. I might miss her struggle, the clues she has laid out that can be picked up by listening for a missing discourse of desire.

IV. IMPLICATIONS FOR PSYCHOTHERAPY

Sharon Thompson made an observation about a small group of adolescent girls among the 400 she has interviewed whom she calls "pleasure narrators" (Thompson, 1990), who describe their own desire and pleasure as key aspects of their first experiences of sexual intercourse. Unlike the majority of the girls with whom she spoke, these girls had talked with their mothers about female sexual desire and pleasure. These mothers interrupted the culture's missing discourse of desire and shared with their daughters what they knew about the sexual feelings their daughters would be experiencing, and in that way validated and celebrated this embodied knowledge. As an adult woman in a relationship with Pamela, listening to her story, I might ask her about her own bodily feelings. Should I wonder with her about the conundrum in which she may find herself: How is it possible for her to know, respond to or speak about her sexual feelings? Should I speak to her about the embodied sexual feelings I experienced when I was her age? Should I introduce to her the possibility of resisting the cultural messages that deny these feelings, the possibility of an embodied discourse of desire? Should I acknowledge that this missing discourse is problematic and engage in resistance against it with her? Would it be possible for me to engage in this same resistance myself? If I could, she and I could try to move towards a way of talking about adolescent girls' and women's sexuality together that takes as central strong sexual feelings, and we might begin to work through the dilemma that these feelings create.

I realize that when girls know, experience and speak about those fabulous feelings in their bodies, trouble follows – for them and for their parents, teachers and therapists. Girls' sexual desire upsets people, because it challenges and might upset the cultural mandate which requires that girls (and women) not be connected to their bodies in general, and to their sexual hunger in particular. Girls' sexual desire is an interruption of the condoned version of what happens in girls' bodies. If girls know their desire, what else might they begin to know about themselves and their situation in the culture?

ENDNOTES

1. See Miller and Simon (1980) for a summary of Erikson's, Piaget's and Kohlberg's disembodied descriptions of sexuality in adolescence.

2. This young woman was a participant in a study of adolescents considered at-risk for school leaving and early pregnancy or parenting funded by the Boston Foundation, with additional support from the Mailman Foundation.

REFERENCES

Brown, L. (Ed.). (1988). *A guide to reading narratives of moral conflict and choice for self and moral orientation.* (Monograph No. 2). Cambridge, MA: Harvard Project on the Psychology of Women and the Development of Girls, Harvard Graduate School of Education.

Brown, L., Debold, E., Tappan, M. & Gilligan, C. (in press). Reading narratives of conflict for self and moral voice: A relational method. In W. Kurtines and J. Gewirtz (Eds.). *Handbook of moral behavior and development: Theory, research and application.* Hillsdale, NJ: Lawrence Erlbaum.

Brown, L. M. & Gilligan, C. (1990, August). *Listening for self and relational voices: A responsive/resisting readers guide.* Paper presented at the annual meeting of the American Psychological Association, Boston, MA.

Cixous, H. (1981). The laugh of the Medusa. In E. Marks and I. de Courtivron (Eds.). *New French Feminisms.* New York: Schocken.

Chodorow, N. (1974). *The reproduction of mothering: Psychoanalysis and the psychology of gender.* Berkeley, CA: University of California Press.

Chodorow, N. (1989). *Feminism and psychoanalytic theory.* New Haven, CT: Yale University Press.

Coles, R. (1985). Introduction. In R. Coles & G. Stokes. *Sex and the American teenager.* New York: Harper Colophon Books.

Dallery, A. (1989). The politics of writing (the) body: *Ecriture feminine.* In A. Jaggar and S. Bordo (Eds.), *Gender/body/Knowledge.* New Brunswick, NJ: Rutgers University Press.

Dalsimer, K. (1986). *Female adolescence: Psychoanalytic reflections on works of literature.* New Haven: Yale University Press.

deMonteflores, C. & Schultz, S. J. (1978). Coming out: Similarities and differences for lesbians and gay men. *Journal of Social Issues, 34*(3), 59-72.

Duggan, L. (1990). From instincts to politics: Writing the history of sexuality in the U.S. *Journal of Sex Research, 27*(1), 95-112.

Espin, O. (1984). Cultural and historical influences on sexuality in Hispanic/Latin women: Implications for psychotherapy. In C. Vance (Ed.), *Pleasure and danger: Exploring female sexuality.* Boston: Routledge and Kegan Paul.

Fine, M. (1988). Sexuality, schooling and adolescent females: The missing discourse of desire. *Harvard Educational Review, 58*(1), 29-53.

Foucault, M. (1978). *The history of sexuality, Volume 1: An introduction.* New York: Vintage.

Gilligan, C. (1977). Woman's place in man's lifecycle. *Harvard Educational Review, 49*(4), 431-446.

Gilligan, C. (1982). *In a different voice: Psychological theory and women's development.* Cambridge: Harvard University Press.

Gilligan, C. (1990). Joining the resistance: Psychology, politics, girls and women. *Michigan Quarterly Review, 29*(4), 501-536.

Gilligan, C, Brown, L., & Rogers, A. (1990). Psyche embedded: A place for body, relationships and culture in personality theory. In A. Rabin et al. (Eds.). *Studying persons and lives*. New York: Springer.

Hite, S. (1976). *The Hite report: A nationwide study of female sexuality*. New York: Dell Publishing Company.

Irigaray, L. (1981). This sex which is not one. In E. Marks and I. de Courtivron (Eds.), *New French Feminisms*. New York: Schocken.

Irigaray, L. (1985). *This sex which is not one*. Ithaca, NY: Cornell University Press.

Jordan, J. (1987). Clarity in connection: Empathic knowing, desire and sexuality. *Work in progress* No. 29. Wellesley, MA: Stone Center Working Papers Series.

Kaplan, L. (1990). *The dynamics of desire: Early sexual abuse and adult sexual desire*. Unpublished doctoral dissertation, Massachusetts School of Professional Psychology, Dedham, MA.

Llera, D. (1991). *Sexually abused adolescent females: Preventing victimization by introducing desire*. Unpublished manuscript, Harvard University.

Miller, J. B. (1976). *Toward a new psychology of women*. Boston: Beacon Press.

Miller, P. and Simon, W. (1980). The development of sexuality in adolescence. In J. Adelsen, (Ed.), *Handbook of adolescent psychology*. New York: J. Wiley and Sons.

Miller, J. B. (1984). The development of women's sense of self. *Work in progress*, No. 12. Wellesley, MA: Stone Center Working Papers Series.

Rogers, A. & Gilligan, C. (1988). *The language of adolescent girls: Themes of moral voice and stages of ego development*. (Monograph No. 6). Cambridge, MA: Harvard Project on the Psychology of Women and The Development of Girls, Harvard Graduate School of Education.

Rubin, G. (1984). Thinking sex: Notes for a radical theory of the politics of sexuality. In C. Vance (Ed.), *Pleasure and danger: Exploring female sexuality*. Boston: Routledge and Kegan Paul.

Snitow, A., Stansell, C. & Thompson, S. (Eds.). (1983). *Powers of desire: The politics of sexuality*. New York: Monthly Review Press.

Surrey, J. (1984). The "self-in-relation:" A theory of women's development. *Work in progress*, No. 13. Wellesley, MA: Stone Center Working Papers Series.

Thompson, S. (1984). Search for tomorrow: On feminism and the reconstruction of teen romance. In C. Vance (Ed.). *Pleasure and danger: Exploring female sexuality*. Boston: Routledge and Kegan Paul.

Thompson, S. (1990). Putting a big thing in a little hole: Teenage girls' accounts of sexual initiation. *Journal of Sex Research, 27*(3), 341-351.

Tolman, D. (1990). *Discourses of adolescent girls' sexual desire in developmental psychology and feminist scholarship*. Unpublished manuscript, Harvard University.

Vance, C. (Ed.). (1984). *Pleasure and danger: Exploring female sexuality*. Boston: Routledge and Kegan Paul.

SECTION II: STRATEGIES OF RESISTANCE

Telling a Girl's Life: Self-Authorization as a Form of Resistance

Lyn Mikel Brown

What would it mean for a girl at the edge of adolescence to tell the truth about her life, to speak honestly and openly about her experiences? What would she say if she were to talk to another about her thoughts and feelings – about herself and the world of relationships she engages on a daily basis – about what she sees and

Lyn Mikel Brown, EdD, is Assistant Professor of Education at Colby College and a member of the Harvard Project on the Psychology of Women and the Development of Girls. Her work focuses on girls' psychological development, girls' education, and feminist methods. She is currently writing a book with Carol Gilligan on a five-year collaborative relationship among a group of researchers, girls, and women teachers.

Preparation of this paper was supported by grants from the Cleveland Foundation, the George Gund Foundation, the Lilly Endowment, and the Spencer Foundation. An early version of this paper was presented in R. Ochberg and M. Gergen (Chairs), *The gender politics of narrative: Women's and men's life stories*, a symposium conducted at the 98th Annual Meeting of the American Psychological Association, Boston, MA.

hears around her; about her fears, her anger, her confusion, her ambivalence; about her power, her hopes, her desires, her fantasies? In this paper I suggest that for a girl to speak about such things in this culture at this time would be, as Nancy K. Miller (1988) suggests, "to protest against the available fiction of female becoming" (p. 129), to refuse the established story of a woman's life, to avoid what Carolyn Heilbrun (1988) terms "female impersonation" (p. 126).

A girl who chooses to authorize her life experiences by speaking openly about them resists the security of convention and moves into uncharted territory; she sets herself adrift, disconnects from the mainland; she risks being, for a time, storyless. And to be without a story - to be without the conventional story of female becoming – can be a deeply frightening experience, since it is to be without a model and thus potentially to be on one's own, confronting the responsibility for authoring one's life. As Carolyn Heilbrun (1988) reminds us in *Writing a Woman's Life:*

> [I]t is a hard thing to make up stories to live by. We can only retell and live by the stories we have read or heard. We live our lives through texts. They may be read, or chanted, or experienced electronically, or come to us, like the murmurings of our mothers, telling us what conventions demand. Whatever their form or medium, these stories have formed us all; they are what we must use to make new fictions, new narratives. (p. 37)

What would it mean for a girl – against the stories read, chanted, or murmured to her – to choose to tell the truth of her life aloud to another person at the very point when she is invited into the larger cultural story of womanhood – that is, at early adolescence? Centrally, this is a question about relationship; about a girl's relationship to the culture and about her relationship to someone she can trust will listen. To whom would a girl speak and in what context? Who would listen to the story she dares to author? What does she risk in the telling?

To answer such questions it would seem we need to ask who was this adolescent girl as a child and what has she to lose or gain from speaking about what she knows about herself and her relationships, what she feels and thinks, what she knows from experience. Listening to young girls, I suggest, is the only way to fully understand the nature of the choice a girl at the edge of adolescence makes about what story to tell about her life.

My colleagues and I have identified a pattern of voices we have heard when we listen to the interview-narratives of young girls over time, as they move from childhood to the edge of adolescence (see Brown, 1989; Brown & Gilligan, 1990; Gilligan, 1990a, 1990b; Rogers & Gilligan, 1988). Listening at one year intervals to the stories girls tell about themselves and their relationships; using an interpretive method – a guide to reading or listening to narratives for self and relational voices – we have witnessed girls shift from engagement in a rich social world of childhood, in which thoughts and feelings – both good and bad – are spoken about directly and publicly, to a struggle at the edge of adolescence to hold on to what they feel and think and therefore know, to authorize their experiences, and not to replace real with inauthentic or idealized relationships. These girls score highly on standard measures of social and personality development – yet when we listen to the way they speak about themselves and their relationships in interview narratives they show evidence of loss, struggle, and signs of an impasse in their ability to act in the face of conflict.

To highlight this pattern I begin with eight-year-old Jesse, whose voice resonates with other girls her age we have talked with.[1] Jesse at eight is both somewhat shy and boldly expressive; she is direct, has strong feelings – both good and bad – and has a sense of her own authority. What can we learn if we begin with Jesse and follow her as she moves from one year to the next? What will Jesse come to know about herself and her relationships over time? And what will Jesse's knowledge and experience suggest about girls experience at the edge of adolescence?

Jesse describes a social world in which feelings are spoken about directly. She is quick to point out that in this world people can be hurt greatly by whispering, telling secrets, poking fun; just as people can be responsive and loving, they can also be thoughtless and cruel. In her eight-year-old world, it is common to be talked about publicly, to find oneself the topic of heated debate.

Yet, Jesse is by no means a hapless victim. She engages fully and publicly in this social drama. She tends to speak of her thoughts and feelings in direct ways, willing to acknowledge and speak out to others with whom she is in relationship about bad or hurt feelings, anger, resentment or frustration, as well as feelings of love, fondness, and loyalty. She tells stories of times when she refuses to take "no" for an answer. If she thinks someone is not listening, she will try again, and if that doesn't work, she sometimes finds creative, even disruptive, ways to be heard.

At eight, for example, Jesse talks about her feelings when "sometimes my friends have friends over when I'm playing with them and I feel left out." Such exclusive treatment is unfair, she says, "Because you should like all your friends together. If you had a friend over, you shouldn't just play with one and leave the other one out . . . and feeling down and out of the game." What could she do to make things different, the interviewer wants to know?

> I would just go over to them, and go in the other friend's ear, I would kind of take them over somewhere else where the other of her friends couldn't hear, and I would say, "This is really making me feel bad, for leaving me out. Can you please play with me too?" That "I will go home if you don't, cause this isn't any fun for me, just sitting here."
>
> HAVE YOU TRIED THAT?
>
> Yeah, but one friend just said, "Just go home."
>
> WHEN THAT HAPPENS . . . DO YOU CONTINUE TO PLAY WITH THEM ANYWAY? OR DO YOU SAY . . .
>
> They don't really care, they don't really care. They just leave – they just don't talk to me. They whisper in each other's ear, saying things about me. I just don't like it.

Jesse does go home but she does not let the issue rest. "It takes me a couple of weeks to understand it," she says, but in time she devises an elaborate plan to show her friend how she felt, at the time in order to make them "even." In the end, she explains, "I would have a friend over and also have her over. . . . I would show her how I felt." For Jesse being "even" meant her friend would have to know and understand the hurt she felt. This knowledge was, necessary for their relationship to continue. "If we're even, she says – meaning the friend knows what Jesse knows about exclusion and abandonment - "then we could start being friends again."

People, Jesse says at eight, "have different feelings." Jesse's awareness that people are different, that they may disagree and, as a result, sometimes people get hurt, is evident as she responds to a common problem of relational conflict posed in the form of an Aesop's Fable – a story about a large and stubborn porcupine who has been invited to spend the winter by a family of well-intentioned moles, who then discover that living with a porcupine is essentially unbearable[2]–Jesse says, "the mole is asking him to leave, but the porcupine doesn't want to, because the porcupine is comfortable; but he keeps on forcing him and [the mole] keeps on saying "no." "Porcupines and moles," Jesse decides, "shouldn't be together because they make a really bad combination." And so it would be best, she decides, to make the cave larger and to "make bigger paths" for the animals to walk. This would make the animals happy and the forest "settled" but would not dissolve the differences between the animals: "They could make their own tracks, she concludes, "they could make their own paths."

A full year later, at nine, Jesse returns to the story of the porcupine and moles. She now begins to speak about what she thinks and feels in different voices, voices that co-exist but do not at this time speak directly to each other: In one voice Jesse says she would have the moles say to the porcupine, "I'm sorry, but please get out. This is my house. I'm not going to let you in anymore, so leave." And then, in another quite different voice, she ponders the situation: "It's the only shelter they have. If it's snowy they would be so cold and they would freeze . . . and they can have a hole to be warm in . . . it's like having a baby in your house."

Thus Jesse's world is one of complicated feelings. A prism of feelings – from anger and feeling wretched to love and warmth, like having a baby in the house – a world of emotions that has a sense of edge and color and distinction. She holds all these feelings, moving from one to the next, speaking in one voice then another. Along with these voices we hear what sound like disembodied lines from parents and teachers that drop into Jesse's ears and into her world about what to know and what not to know, what to say and what not to say: "Communicating is better than fighting," Jesse says, referring to the porcupine and the moles, and with this blanket statement the complexity of what she has felt and thought about their differences seems to dissolve. In the end, she summarizes, "You should be nice to your friends and communicate with them and not . . . do what you want." And her wish for the porcupine and moles is that they "are happy and they don t have to fight anymore. They could just be friends and they could stay like that forever.

But despite this ideal vision, which covers over strong feelings and earlier distinctions, conflict and disagreement are commonplace in Jesse's relationships; part and parcel of the ordinary. Jesse marks the uneventful dailiness of conflict when she says of herself and her best friend in third grade, "we usually get in fights, because she wants to do one thing and we don't know what to do and we get all bored. And then finally she goes, are we friends? So we are and we try to find something to do."

Jesse has changed in subtle ways between second and third grades. As one might guess, she is more articulate – she describes her thoughts and feelings more vividly. Yet, there is an emerging awareness of the knowledge and the danger in authentic encounters; in "real" relationships. Having taken in the message "cooperating is better than fighting," Jesse begins to equate fighting with trouble from authorities, with anger, meanness, and noise, and cooperating with praise, niceness, calmness, and quiet; she is, it seems, undergoing a bit of ear and voice-training. Though she claims that people "can keep their different ideas and . . . still be friends," she struggles with disagreement, recognizing early the dangers in speaking directly or expressing anger. Jesse is now sometimes willing to be nice to make the relationship "calm" and her friends happy so they will play with her, rather than because she feels like being nice." Cooperating" in this way is better, she says, because "you don't get into fights and it's just calm and so it is not noisy and you can play." The interviewer asks her to explain:

> WHY DON'T YOU FEEL GOOD ABOUT [GETTING INTO FIGHTS]?
>
> That you are losing a friend and that you are both unhappy.

IF YOU SAID, "NO." TO HER, "I DON'T WANT TO DO THAT," WOULD YOU RISK LOSING HER?

Yah.

HOW DO YOU KNOW THAT SHE MIGHT GO AWAY?

Because she always, well, I am not going to lose her for a long time, because always the next day at school we hug and say we are ready and say hi, because we both forget about it. I think I would lose her because she's very easy to lose, you know. If I say no and I walked out the door, she would come and drag me in again and she would start screaming at me. And she would start crying and I don't want that to happen.

The irony of this story, it seems, is that Jesse has not described a friend who is "easy to lose" at all. In fact, if Jesse *were* to say no, her friend would not let her go; "she would come and drag" Jesse in the room again, and "start screaming" at her. Jesse, it seems, has presented the most authentic and gripping scene of relationship yet, and has almost in the same breath ruled it out as an example of relationship at all. Yet, at the same time, one can understand her fear. The risk is real and substantial to her. Losing a friend is "horrible," Jesse says, "because you wouldn't have a best friend to play with all the time . . . and I don't think you could find a friend just like that person."

Indeed, at ten, Jesse is consumed with what is and is not a relationship. Her strong feelings, spoken directly and with passion, can be dangerous since they are disruptive. Signs of disruption–anger and noise, getting riled up and anxious – are cause for being "ignored," left out, abandoned. Repeatedly Jesse speaks about her discomfort with anger, with noise, with yelling and the value of "talking quietly," of being "calm," and of dealing with disagreements in private. This is a good way to handle disagreements, she says, "because it doesn't get anybody mad . . . everybody doesn't get all riled up . . . so that you are mad for the rest of the day and your mom starts yelling at you because you are so mad and you get anxious and do things you are not supposed to do." From such situations, Jesse says, "I learn to agree with people . . . and don't get nervous and all riled up because it will just start more trouble."

And so what once were the signs of authentic relationship for Jesse, the possibility of feeling another's pain as well as joy, and the potential for difference and disagreement, are now withdrawn as too dangerous and risky.

Jesse, now eleven and in the fifth grade, responds to the Porcupine and Moles fable. At eight, you may recall, Jesse considered that perhaps the moles and porcupine were "a bad combination." At eleven, Jesse wishes to make the hole bigger because "it would be nice to have a neighbor in the house." It would be possible, she says for the moles to say to the porcupine, "'I really don't want you here . . . ' and tell him to get out," but that would not be "a nice way to do it . . . because the porcupine would feel left out." What sounded like advice from adults at nine: "compromise is better than fighting," is replaced by a stronger message with a similar ring: "always be nice to a friend." Unlike her self at eight and nine, Jesse at eleven no longer mentions the moles' discomfort as they were stuck by the porcupine's sharp quills, but focuses only on the porcupine's loneliness and hurt feelings. The moles no longer say "no" to hurt or inattentiveness; they do not confront the porcupine directly or disrupt the "nice" scene with any sense of anger or indignation. Differences and potential conflict between these animals who once "made their own tracks" is now covered over by a sole concern for niceness and neighborliness as prerequisites for friendship.

Speaking up about her feelings, no problem at all for Jesse at eight, and of some concern for her at nine, is now, at eleven, the basis for real trepidation. If a girl doesn't like another girl, Jesse says, she "should pretend that [she] likes her." The source of this new fear is the "perfect girl" – the girl who has no bad thoughts or feelings, the kind of person everyone wants to be with; the girl who, in her perfection, is worthy of real praise and attention, worthy of inclusion and love. Jesse describes her as the girl who is "so good in math." She is the girl who speaks quietly, calmly, who is always nice and kind, never mean or bossy. The girl, Jesse implies, she wished she could say she hates. And sometimes, Jesse says, "your attitude just goes bonkers because you are really jealous of [her]."

In the presence of the perfect girl, Jesse, who has strong feelings, who says, "Sometimes I have to just get my anger out of me," cannot speak, since strong feelings, spoken or acted on, carry severe consequences. Saying the wrong thing or saying something in the wrong way, Jesse says, is "terrifying." Asked to tell about a time when she wanted to say something but didn't, Jesse says:

> When you are really mad at somebody and you want to say something really bad, but you can't, you just can't. It's like it comes out of your mouth and you forget what you are going to say . . . or I don't say something because . . . somebody says a real good idea and everybody agrees and mine is like the exact opposite and you don't want everybody to leave you out and say, "Oh, that's horrible! Why, we don't want to do that." Because you sort of feel bad when that happens.
>
> CAN YOU SAY MORE ABOUT THAT?
>
> Sometimes when you have friends and they are being real nice to you and you are trying to be nice to them and usually when you are nice to them, they are nice to you and sometimes when other people say something that everybody likes, and they say, "Oh, that's a good idea," and you have the exact opposite, you feel like "Oh oh, they really won't want me to do this, or they won't want me in the club since I don't have good ideas," and you sort of get afraid to say it. And sometimes you get afraid to say things like "I hate you" when you're mad at somebody.
>
> WHY ARE YOU AFRAID TO SAY THAT?
>
> Because a lot of times they get really mad and it really terrifies you because you feel like they are going to tell somebody and they are going to get almost the whole class on her side and it would be one against, I don't know, ten.
>
> IN THOSE SITUATIONS, HOW DO YOU FEEL?
>
> I don't feel very good. I feel like I'm making this whole fight, that it is really turning out to be a mess.

Jesse's choice to speak will upset the precarious "nice and polite" scene with her friends; will, in fact, reveal it as a false scene since people will not be nice to her if she is not nice to them, that is, if she says what she thinks. This gives her "a weird feeling," makes her "confused sort of," and "really terrifies" her. Jesse, who at eight would tell her friend "this is making me feel bad, I'm going home," is now at eleven "afraid to say" what she thinks and "terrified" of what might happen if she says what she feels.

Thus, what seemed matter of fact, ordinary life to Jesse at eight – people play and people get angry, they have strong feelings; people wish to speak and expect to be heard – has become momentous to Jesse at eleven. Faced with the potential to "upset the whole class" and afraid of being ignored, embarrassed, ridiculed, Jesse carefully chooses when to speak. Talking about a time when "a whole group of friends are mad at one of my really good friends," Jesse illustrates the conflict other girls describe between speaking up or choosing to remain silent. If she chooses to stay out of the disagreement, Jesse risks herself and her feelings. She says, "I usually just stay away and I know how I act when that happens, I can tell. . . . I am not really me. I can tell when it's not really [me]." On the other hand, if she stays with herself and her feelings and gets involved in public confrontation she risks the "terrifying" feelings of starting fights she cannot stop. When can Jesse afford to stay with herself and speak? When should she distance herself and "stay out of it," "forget it," choose to "agree" for the sake of relationships with others? Like other girls her age,[3] at the edge of adolescence, Jesse shows an emerging propensity to separate what she knows and loves from what she believes she ought to do in order to be seen as cooperative, kind, and good – the kind of girl others, she thinks, want to be with. If she stays with what she wants and says what she thinks, she fears she may be the cause of social chaos, abandoned by others in her undesirable feelings, her imperfection. If she "pretends" and "agrees" and is nice when she does not feel nice, she abandons herself, her thoughts and feelings and becomes, as Jesse says, "not really me."

Jesse seems caught between speaking about what she knows about relationships – a knowledge gained from looking and listening – and increased pressure to negate this knowledge for an idealized and fraudulent view of herself and her relationships – the view carried by the image of the perfect girl. In a world of cliques and in-groups, the image of the perfect girl is powerful – being her can assure Jesse of inclusion, love, attention. The terrifying or terrorizing nature of this image lies in its power to encourage Jesse to give over the reality of her astute observations of herself and the human world around her – or at least to modulate her voice and not speak about what she sees and hears, feels and thinks, and therefore knows. Voice-training by adults, especially adult "good women," reinforces these images of female perfection – "nice girls" are always calm, controlled, quiet; they never cause a ruckus, they are never noisy, bossy, or aggressive, they are not anxious and do not cause trouble.

And so Jesse, at the brink of young womanhood, is consumed with what is and what is not a relationship, with the distinction between what she knows from experience and what is taken increasingly by girls and by the adults around her to be reality. This impending division leads her to pay close attention and to describe the relational world like a naturalist, carefully portraying the changes caused by her every move, revealing with remarkable clarity the motives and intentions and perspectives of others, and also listening to the way this world is named and described. The model of the perfect girl threatens to keep Jesse from seeing what she is looking at and listening to what she is hearing. Thus, while Jesse is more subtle, having become cognitively more sophisticated in her understanding of herself and the social world over time, she is also more cautious, more aware of what it means to know what she knows, more willing to silence herself rather than to risk loss of relationships and public disagreement.

Listening to Jesse reminds us that long before a girl reaches adolescence she hears both directly and indirectly the established story of the good woman. We hear Jesse as young as eight and nine speak of the dangers – exclusion, abandonment, ridicule – of expressing strong feelings such as anger; we listen as, over time, she takes in the conventional equation of female directness and lucidity with rudeness and trouble; how she silences herself, forgets what she wants to say rather than to risk public disruption; and how her understandable frustration at the perfect girl image is taken over by jealousy as she accepts the romantic promise of idealized relationships in store only for those who are always kind and nice. And we see, with these changes over time, an emerging split between what

Jesse sees and hears, what she knows from experience, and what is so-called reality. It is not unreasonable to assume that Jesse, like other adolescent girls my colleagues and I have spoken with, will look back at her childhood clarity – her direct expressions of anger as well as her playfulness and pleasure in relationships – with embarrassment and dismay, as a time of rudeness or childish immaturity she has, with a mix of natural growth and social discipline, outgrown.

Carolyn Heilbrun (1988) suggests that for women "the last third of life is likely to require new attitudes and new courage" (p. 124). "It is perhaps only in old age, certainly past fifty," she remarks, "that women can stop being female impersonators (p. 126). . . . once [they have] moved beyond the categories our available narratives have provided for women" (p. 131). Sara Ruddick (1990), pondering women's move "from maternal thinking to peace politics," speaks in a similar way of the need for women to become lucid, to see and name, and therefore become responsible for the pain they and others suffer at the hand of oppressive authorities. Ruddick, concerned with what prevents mothers "from seeing, let alone caring about the pain of distant or different others" (p. 16), with what allows them to "protect themselves from lucidity and therefore from responsibility" (p. 17), and how to "shift the balance . . . from denial to lucid knowledge" (p. 20), speaks of the necessity of acquiring a feminist consciousness that allows women to name the impact of conventional gender stereotypes. She says:

> They come to recognize that the stories they have been told and tell themselves about what it means "to be a woman" are mystifying and destructive . . . In unravelling these . . . stories, mothers acquiring feminist consciousness may well be prompted to explore undefensively their ambitions and sexual desires and in particular to describe realistically the angers and ambivalences of maternal love. . . . Hitherto silenced voices, edging toward lucid speech, are developing voices, transformed by new experiences of seeing and saying. (pp. 21-23)

Like Mary Belenky, Blythe Clinchy, Nancy Goldberger, and Jill Tarule in their book *Women's Ways of Knowing* (1986) both

Heilbrun and Ruddick mark a developmental progression in women's lives from an acceptance of– or at least a nondisruptive silence about – the conventions of female goodness, to a critical feminist consciousness – a "way of knowing" that is aware, reflective, that seeks to name oppressive authority, that comes to a lucidity and public outspokenness about life circumstances and thus leads to the possibility for constructing a different way of being in the world with others. But Jesse's voice at eight and nine and ten, and the voices of other young girls I have talked with, raise questions about whether the lucidity women find or gain or develop in later life is not in fact a lucidity they once had, then lost, and have since refound or recovered; whether women in later life create entirely "*new* experiences of seeing or saying" or "require *new* attitudes and *new* courage," or whether they recall earlier, older, familiar experiences, attitudes, and courage – experiences that, for a time, for safety's sake, they forgot, denied or repressed.[4] Was there a time when we, as women, once saw clearly what we were looking at and named, in the face of conflict, our strong feelings about the complicated and rich world of relationships we engaged? If so, when and how was this clarity of vision lost? At what cost?

For girls in this culture at this time, adolescence appears to mark a potential point of departure from life experience. Adolescence itself is a time when a variety of perspectives can be held and coordinated, a time when the hypothetical and the abstract can be entertained. Thus adolescents come face to face with alternative possibilities, with the potential for conflict and choice. And with the ability to abstract comes the rewards and dangers of the capacity to separate what one knows from experience from other possible scenarios. For girls, adolescence is a time of particular vulnerability; a point where a girl is encouraged to give over or to disregard or devalue what she feels and thinks – what she knows about the world of relationships – if she is to enter the dominant views of conventional womanhood. Wooed by idealized relationships, by the possibility of perfection and purity, and by the new image of the superwoman – the woman who has it all with no outward signs of distress or struggle – she is encouraged to enter, to buy into, a story that she has not known to be true from her experiences in childhood. For a girl to do otherwise, to tell a different story true to her rich and varied experiences of childhood relationship – to stay with what she knows in the face of pressure to not know – would be to engage in an act of resistance, an act of moral courage in the face of potential risk to her body and her psyche.

In listening to girls poised at the edge of adolescence I hear them speak of their confusion and their fight, their struggle for understanding. They reveal a great desire to be heard, to be in authentic relationships – relationships in which both people can speak about what they most passionately feel and know with a sense of personal authority. They struggle "to make [others] understand"; they reveal their desire to be heard, they "hunt down," in one girl's words, those they feel must understand them for relationships to survive.

While, as Jesse reminds us, the division between the rich complexity of felt experience and the narrow but rewarded established conventions of femininity is forged throughout female childhood, at the edge of adolescence – at ten and eleven and twelve – girls seem to struggle most passionately to authorize their life experiences, to tell their own stories, to hold on to what they know. Sometimes consciously and sometimes not, they name the fear, the vulnerability, the anxiety they feel in the face of those who will not listen or who use their power to impart a message of false relationships. In the face of the confusion this division imparts, they seek the presence of someone who will listen in order to give their knowledge a space and a legitimacy. To be an authority on their own experience requires another person who will acknowledge them as such, not simply an audience but a relationship in which they are taken seriously.

Jesse at eight, who spoke to others directly, with candor, who revealed her strong feelings about love and hate with hope for understanding and response, struggles at ten and eleven with the terrorizing messages of female goodness. She cannot alone "protest against the available fiction of female becoming," she cannot all by herself resist "female impersonation." To do so requires not that she alone makes available alternative texts or stories, but that new stories about relationships between women and between girls and women – mothers, therapists, teachers – be created. Telling a girl's life as a life about knowing and persistence – telling an intriguing, interesting story, with passion and political awareness – is an act of resistance that requires no small measure of bravery. In the telling a girl authorizes her story and a woman, if she can remain in the girl's presence and, in the terms of Adrienne Rich (1979), be a "witness in her defense," may recover a story long forgotten.

ENDNOTES

1. Jesse is a participant in a five-year longitudinal study of girls' development conducted at the Laurel School for Girls in Cleveland, Ohio. Specifically, Jesse is part of a group of 20 second grade girls – eight year olds, most of them white and middle-class – who we interviewed once a year for five years, until they turned twelve. In large part, this analysis of Jesse has been excerpted from an earlier page entitled "The Psychology of Women and the Development of Girls" written by myself and Carol Gilligan (1990).

2. This adaptation of Aesop's Fables to listen to how children and adolescents solve relational conflicts was designed by Kay Johnston (1988).

3. Though by this I mean, specifically, other girls in the project in which Jesse has participated, recent evidence suggests that adolescent girls from different ethnic and socioeconomic backgrounds also struggle with ideals of purity and perfection, often in the form of the Madonna-whore myth (Taylor & Ward, in press).

4. Annie Rogers and Carol Gilligan (1988) have raised this question in their analysis of girls' responses to sentence stems. See also Emily Hancock's (1989) book *The girl within.* Based on interviews with adult women Hancock suggests that 'reclaiming the authentic identity she'd embodied as a girl" (p. 4) "appears to be key to women's identity" (p. 25).

REFERENCES

Belenky, M., Clinchy, B., Goldberger, N., & Tarule, J. (1986). *Women's ways of knowing*. New York: Basic Books.

Brown, L. (1989). *Narratives of relationship: The development of a care voice in girls ages 7 to 16.* Unpublished doctoral dissertation. Harvard University.

Brown, L. and Gilligan, C. (1990, March). *The psychology of women and the development of girls.* Paper presented at the biannual meeting of the Society for Research on Adolescence, Atlanta, GA.

Gilligan, C. (1990a). Joining the resistance: Psychology, politics, girls and women. *Michigan Quarterly Review, 29*(4), 501-536.

Gilligan, C. (1990b). Teaching Shakespeare's sister. In. C. Gilligan, N. Lyons, and T. Hanmer (Eds.), *Making connections: The relational worlds of adolescent girls at Emma Willard School.* Cambridge, MA: Harvard University Press.

Hancock, E. (1989). *The girl within.* New York: Fawcett Columbine.

Heilbrun, C. (1988). *Writing a woman's life.* New York: Ballantine.
Johnston, K. (1988). Adolescents' solutions to dilemmas in fables: Two moral orientations – two problem-solving strategies. In C. Gilligan, J. Ward, and J. Taylor (Eds.), *Mapping the moral domain.* Cambridge, MA: Harvard Press.
Miller, N. (1988). *Subject to Change.* New York: Columbia University Press.
Rich, A. (1979). *On lies, secrets, and silence.* New York: W. W. Norton.
Rogers, A & Gilligan, C. (1988). *Translating the language of adolescent girls: Themes of moral voice and stages of ego development* (Monograph No. 6). Cambridge, MA: Project on the Psychology of Women and the Development of Girls, Harvard Graduate School of Education.
Ruddick, S. (1990, February). *From maternal thinking to peace politics.* Paper presented at Women, Girls, and Education lecture series, Harvard Graduate School of Education, Cambridge, MA.
Taylor, J. & Ward, J. (in press). Culture, sexuality, and school: Perspectives from focus groups in six cultural communities. *Women's Studies Quarterly.*

"A Belief in Self Far Greater Than Anyone's Disbelief": Cultivating Resistance Among African American Female Adolescents

Tracy Robinson
Janie Victoria Ward

Within the biography of each individual African American, the convergence of race, gender, and class has its own unique configuration. However, mindful of the particular ways our lives have been shaped as a result of the subordinate status of our race and gender, and as African American women in psychology, we believe that many of the challenges and concerns we have confronted in our passage from childhood to adult status have been largely ignored in traditional social science literature. To this piece on resistance in African American adolescent females we bring not only our scholarly expertise as developmental and educational psychologists, but our reflections upon our own histories of healthy resistance in a society that continually denigrates womanhood and blackness. At various times over our life courses we have had to confront the

Tracy Robinson, EdD, is Assistant Professor in the Department of Counselor Education at North Carolina State University. Her research interest is the convergence of gender with race and ethnicity in psychosocial development.

Janie Victoria Ward, EdD, is Assistant Professor of Education and Human Services at Simmons College. Her research interests include the psychosocial development of adolescents of color, and racial socialization within African American families. She is a member of the Harvard Project on the Psychology of Women and the Development of Girls.

omnipresent and powerful forces poised ready to humiliate, demean and destroy our efforts at racial affirmation and self-determination. As children we resisted various teachers throughout the educational pipeline who did not cultivate our highest educational aspirations. In our professions we continue to resist aligning ourselves with researchers who either ignore the issues and concerns of African American adolescent populations or inappropriately apply them to cultural frameworks that are Eurocentric. Despite the disproportionate representation of black teens in the grim statistics of teen pregnancies, substance abuse and crime, we resist the perspective that the psychosocial experiences of African American teens are inherently disordered and unhealthy. Moving beyond the pathological models, we choose instead to construct new paradigms which, in exploring the intrapsychic and social conditions conducive to the development of healthy psychosocial functioning, uncover and build upon strengths which are cultivated by African American culture. In our effort to identify and inculcate healthy resistance in black adolescent females, we recognize that there is no monolithic black woman to whom we can all refer, no one social class to which we all belong, and no single manner by which black women can (or should) successfully battle the negative forces of oppression which shape their lives. It is our hope that the approach we provide will be empowering to professionals and we encourage our readers, particularly those who work with African American females, to engage in the work of unmasking each woman's individual history of resistance against those who seek to undermine her efforts to gain self determination and achieve personal and racial affirmation.

African American adolescent girls, as their Euroamerican counterparts, are engaged in the process of identity formation and self-creation. During the passage from adolescence to adulthood critical attitudes are formulated, behaviors are adopted and lifestyle choices are made. However, African American adolescent girls are making this passage embedded within a family and a community that is most often negatively impacted by a sociopolitical context framed by racial, gender, and economic oppression. We suggest that an African American female can be consciously prepared for the sociopolitical environment in which she will live by fostering development of a resistance that will provide her with the necessary tools to think critically about herself, the world and her place in it.

Therapists have described African Americans' passive and active resistances to what blacks perceive as intrusive intrapsychic and social interventions undertaken by ill-informed white mental health professionals (Boyd-Franklin, 1989). However, although African American people, particularly women, have become expert developers and appropriators of resistant attitudes and behaviors, we believe that all of these forms of resistance are not always in our best interest. We suggest that while some of the choices African American girls and women make in their daily lives constitute resistance for survival and may well serve the (short-term) interest of individual survival in a hostile and oppressive environment, not all forms of resistance are conducive to our liberation as an African people. Our primary premise is that there is a critical difference between resistance for survival and resistance for liberation. Resistance for liberation – resistance in which black girls and women are encouraged to acknowledge the problems of, and to demand change in, an environment that oppresses them – embodies our desire to create and adopt a "therapy of empowerment" (Fulani, 1988) that supports African American women's transformation into self-conscious agents engaged in battle on their own behalf. As there have been a number of excellent recent discussions of clinical problems unique to the black adolescent,[1] we will not review specific psychological disorders or therapeutic interventions in this paper. instead, we will elaborate on what we mean by 'resistance for survival' and 'resistance for liberation.' We will identify those potentially destructive elements of the sociocultural environment that young African American women may choose as strategies of resistance for survival: self-denigration due to the internalization of negative self images, excessive autonomy and individualism at the expense of connectedness to the collective, and resistance to "quick fixes" such as early and unplanned pregnancies, substance abuse, school failure and food addictions. We believe that African American girls need to be encouraged to engage in resistance for liberation by avoiding these short term solutions as they erode self-confidence, lower self-esteem, and impair positive identity development. While we contend that the process of growing up necessitates for all black females the engagement of resistant strategies, the examples presented will illustrate what we are proposing as a critical distinction between these strategies. We believe that while forms of resistance undertaken solely to maintain survival can represent dysfunctional adaptations to an oppressive reality and tend only to provide short term relief, efforts of resistance taken up to promote the liberation of one's self and one's community require and sustain a self-conscious process of seeking to identify and transcend imposed systemic barriers by drawing upon the strengths of one's history and cultural connections.

RESISTANCE TO NEGATIVE IMAGES OF THE SELF

Recent studies of preschoolers demonstrate that by age three and four, children of different races are keenly aware that, in this society, white skin color is valued and preferred (Hopson & Hopson, 1988). Television, the prime socializer of Americans, has a long history of negatively depicting both African American individuals and families, and it continues to exclude their representation in most mainstream portrayals of professional vocations. The relentless perpetuation of these negative images, and the exclusionary practices of the media, largely shape the attitudes which white America holds about blacks, as well as the attitudes blacks hold about themselves. As narrow, primarily Eurocentric conceptions of beauty are promoted and socially rewarded; many African American girls struggle to accept their own dark skin and naturally kinky hair as beautiful (Okazawa-Rey, Robinson, & Ward, 1987). When they are not ignored in the media, black adolescent females are usually maligned. The single, most frequent representation of African American adolescent women is the teen mother, who is generally depicted as a low-income future welfare recipient with minimal education and few transferable skills for the work place. She is assumed to be sexually irresponsible and emotionally bankrupt, and thus easily manipulated by the men in her life. The viewer is seldom encouraged to consider the role of external sociopolitical and economic forces on her life and is thus led to conclude that she holds primary responsibility for her limited future options.

This debasing stereotype of adolescent black females is a contemporary representation of the demeaning images that have been employed historically to characterize African American women. These symbolic depictions serve to foster contempt from others and from the self and contribute to some black women's desire to escape psychologically. The result of exposure to negative images of blacks is illustrated by the recollections of Linda, a black adolescent high school sophomore.[2]

> When I'm watching tv, stuff like that, I associated blacks with welfare and stuff like that and it's really bad but . . . when we used to drive through the bad parts of town or something, I would always see blacks out there and (think) I can't be a part of that, that's not me.

In her attempt to distance herself from "those blacks out there," Linda demonstrates an unwillingness to identify with those she has been socialized to denigrate. Her psychological retreat is a survival strategy – an attempt to maintain a positive sense of self amid the onslaught of injurious attacks against African Americans and her culture. However, Linda's survival strategy of cultural disassociation through psychological separation is essentially a posture of subordination, one that places her healthy racial and individual identity development at risk and leaves her vulnerable to the destructive effects of emotional isolation and self-alienation.

For the African American adolescent female, the ability to move beyond the internalization of racial denigration to an internalization of racial pride involves a process of confronting and rejecting oppressive negating evaluations of blackness and femaleness, adopting instead a sense of self that is self-affirming and self-valuing (Collins, 1989; Ladner, 1971; Ward, 1990). To resist in the service of her own liberation, an African American adolescent female must learn to identify negating distortions, understand their origins and whose interests they serve, and must ultimately look beyond these demeaning portrayals by embracing the admirable qualities of black womanhood these images obscure, particularly the unique wisdom, strength and perseverance of African American women. We suggest that Linda needs to establish a positive racial and personal identity through the process of repudiation and affirmation – an act of psychological resistance for liberation – which is perhaps her best defense against the internal and external stresses which threaten to lower her self-esteem and contributes to self-abnegation.

RESISTANCE TO EXCESSIVE INDIVIDUALISM

Conventional theories of adolescence define the teen years as a time of struggle for autonomy and independence (Erikson, 1968). Breaking away from others to find oneself (self discovery) is seen as a marker of maturity, and this privileging of individuality recurs throughout the adolescent psychology literature.

Nobles (1980) and other Afrocentric scholars draw distinctions between EuroAmerican principles of excessive individuality and autonomy and the African worldview where attention is on cooperation and responsibility to the collective. The individual's frame of reference in the African worldview includes an extended definition of the self as "we." Embedded in this "extended self" is the recognition of the individual's connectedness with others. Feminist scholars similarly argue that the desire to maintain and strengthen connections and interdependence between people is an organizing framework by which women develop a sense of self and morality (Gilligan, 1982, Miller, 1976). The discussions of identity construction from Afrocentric and feminist theorists suggest that young African American women, in developing their sense of self-concept, are particularly attuned to issues of human interdependence and collective responsibility.

Adoption of an individualistic ideology is consistent with our highly competitive capitalist society. Along with a steady stream of common socializing messages encouraging autonomy and independence, American teens receive a series of directives advising them how to "make it": "avoid drugs and early sexuality," "stay in school," "get a good job," "resist peer pressure," and "be your own person." Teens hear the dominant achievement ideology that assumes they are ultimately responsible for their own failure and/or success. However, while for many Americans "making it" means achieving the social and financial rewards of middle class status, the subtle message to African American teens suggests the prescription for success for them requires neutralizing or separating from race-allegiances in order to join the white middle class and gain its acceptance. Messages to African American teens which frame failures in achievement as solely "their fault" are inaccurate because the roles of gender, race and class in reward distribution are not acknowledged.

"Racelessness," described by Fordham (1988) as the desire to minimize cultural connections, appears to be a disturbing strategy adopted by some high achieving black students to improve their success in school. To be recognized as bright, articulate and academically successful, these adolescents, fleeing the stigma associated with blackness, are often encouraged to disconnect from their average African American counterparts. Appearing to be raceless is an attempt to counteract the implicit message that says "to be academically successful, you must be white." However, although "acting white" (Fordham & Ogbu, 1986) can be an adaptational survival strategy in the educational arena, it is short term and highly problematic. Racelessness promotes self-alienation and encourages both psychological and physical separation from the broader African American community. The apparent positive relationship between academic success and the belief that such success requires separation from one's culture of origin is disturbing and unfortunate.

It is not our intention to argue that individual effort is not an important ingredient for success or an effective tool against oppression. Instead we are arguing that a value orientation which promotes only individual fulfillment can be detrimental to the African American collective. The image of the self in isolation may situate well with the ideology of individualism and function as resistance for survival, but it works to undermine African American girls' capacity for interpersonal commitment and collective struggle which mark resistance for liberation. This peculiar focus on individuality and separation may make it difficult for African American adolescent females to connect with their shared common destiny with African Americans, a destiny which transcends education and social class, geographic location, sexual orientation and age differences.

Lisa[3] explains,

> If I make it (in the future), I think that the fact that I'm black will be very important because right now I don't think Blacks are doing very well, and I think that whatever Blacks make it have to turn around and help other blacks. Because just the idea of being a people . . . I just think you should care. Because, I mean for a black to make it, someone had to help him. I really don't think there's anything you can do on your own, . . . I mean someone helped you.

Nobles' conception of "the extended self" is seen in the value structure of many black families. Willie (1985) argues that many African American children such as Lisa are encouraged to employ their own personal achievements as a means to resist racism. The importance of hard work and communalism is viewed threefold: as a personal responsibility, as an intergenerational commitment to family, and as a tie to the larger collective. A resistant strategy of liberation, in keeping with African American traditional values, ties individual achievement to collective struggle. We maintain that in the service of personal and cultural liberation, African American adolescent girls must resist an individualism that sees the self as disconnected from others in the black community and, as it is culturally and psychologically dysfunctional, she must resist those who might advocate her isolation and separation from traditional African American cultural practices, values and beliefs.

RESISTANCE TO QUICK FIXES

While the majority of African American teens today are avoiding self-destructive behaviors, black teens continue to be over represented in the juvenile justice system, pregnancy rates are still twice as high among African American teens than whites and heroin and cocaine use are still disproportionately prevalent among African American youths (Gibbs, 1989b). From the perspective of the African American adolescent woman feeling overwhelming despair and hopelessness, employing a "quick fix" to cope with life's exigencies may seem both necessary and pragmatic. For example, in the minds of many young women, becoming a mother is seen as one of the few viable options available to her which might bring real purpose to her life; in circumventing loneliness and disconnection, adolescent pregnancy and parenting can be viewed as an act of resistance to a society that has deemed her of little use and value. Growing numbers of young black women are finding their escape in substance abuse where, at least for a short time, they can anesthetize themselves against the anguish of unemployment, depression, hunger, and powerlessness. Moreover, the increased demand for drugs, coupled with persistent decreases in African American youth employment rates, greatly contributes to the perception that running drugs is a feasible (albeit high risk) employment opportunity.

Researchers estimate that "during the past 15-20 years, obesity has increased 53% among African American adolescents 12-17 years old" (Gortmaker et al., 1987, cited in Desmond et al., 1989, p. 353). We believe that poor nutrition, limited resources for girls' recreational exercise (particularly in urban areas), the use of food to pacify anger and frustration, and an overall lack of knowledge regarding effective methods for changing self-defeating behaviors help to explain this rise in obesity among African American girls. Health care professionals warn that overeating as a "quick fix" in adolescence often causes more serious problems in later life. For example, hypertension and diabetes, two diseases which chronically plague African American women in their later years, are related to or complicated by obesity.

Educational statistics decry the alarming increase in school failure among African American children and adolescents. The numbers of young black women who are academically underachieving, dropping out, or are "kicked and/or pushed out" of our public schools is a scandalous indictment of the system's unwillingness to provide education equitably to all of its children. The choice to leave school prematurely – the "quick fix" of school failure – may in fact be the calculated move of an adolescent who has made a decision for herself that is psychologically empowering. Michelle Fine (1988), in her research on school dropouts, found that in comparison to persisters, dropouts were relatively non-depressed and less willing to mindlessly conform (p. 90). In this light, school failure can be seen as a survival strategy adopted by teens who, feeling bored, devalued and unrecognized, attempt to resist a school system they experience as both disrespectful of, and irrelevant to, their lives. Needless to say, an African American adolescent woman's decision to adopt a strategy of resistance such as school failure or academic underachievement as a means for counteracting the results of ineffective educational practices is disturbingly shortsighted. The disempowering consequences of undereducation can negatively impact black women's ability to think critically, solve problems, and make the self-affirming, informed choices necessary for her economic survival.

Whether it be food addictions, irresponsible sexual behavior and premature pregnancy, or any one of the many ways African American adolescent women choose to endure the consequences of their devaluation, we maintain that adopting any one of the aforementioned "quick fix" survival strategies as a chosen mode of resistance is ultimately unwise, unsafe and uncertain. It is our contention that an African American adolescent woman must foster and be encouraged to form resistant attitudes and behaviors which move beyond temporary relief by contributing to her liberation and empowering her towards self-determination. An African American adolescent woman who has liberation and self-determination on her mind will come to see "quick fixes" for the social and psychological traps that they are and discover instead alternative avenues to personal empowerment and positive change. Adopting such a position is a critical step towards black women's self-validation, affirmation and self-care.

AN AFROCENTRIC MODEL TOWARD RESISTANCE

Throughout this work we have argued that there is a clear demarcation between resistance that is oriented toward survival and resistance that is engaged in the service of liberation. We realize that a myriad of factors contribute to the selection of resistance strategies. However, resistance strategies most frequently adopted by African American girls have been crisis-oriented, short-term strategies, and resistance strategies toward liberation are, regrettably, the exception. Ironically, as we have delineated, those same survival strategies young black women adopt to withstand the assaults of oppression frequently result in abetting their subjugation over time.

The model we propose integrates the socialization of African American adolescent women by addressing gender specific issues and concerns and incorporates an Afrocentric perspective of racial identity and self-determination. Collins' (1989) work on black women's culture suggests that black women value and are empowered by their ability to make use of their subjective knowledge-base to challenge grounded assumptions about the world and their place in it. Referred to by black women as "mother wit," (Luttrell, 1989), this particularistic wisdom upon which they can draw helps them cope with the realities of racism and sexism. Adolescent African American women can be helped to build upon this indigenous source of strength by learning to trust their own voices and perspectives and to develop what bell hooks (in press) calls the black woman's "oppositional gaze:" a way to observe the social world critically and to oppose those ideas and ways of being that are disempowering to the self. African American adolescent females, by being made aware of the historical and contemporary instances of black female resistance, can be empowered through their connection to black women's long history as freedom fighters and social activists.

Oliver (1989) argues that dysfunctional cultural adaptations to structurally induced social pressures are a result of the absence of an Afrocentric world view. This would require that African Americans recognize the presence of racism and understand its profound impact on the economics, culture, family, psyche and spirit of African Americans. Moreover, an Afrocentric world view would encourage African Americans to develop an awareness of African culture and traditions. Resistance oriented toward survival fails to incorporate an Afrocentric view point. We suggest that an Afrocentric model can be central in enabling African American adolescent females to foster resistance for liberation and empowerment.

The Nguzo Saba refers to a value system that African Americans are encouraged to adopt based on traditional African philosophies. The seven principles of the Nguzo Saba include: umoja (unity), kujichagulia (self-determination), ujima (collective work and responsibility), ujaama (cooperative economics), nia (purpose), kuumba (creativity) and imani (faith) (Karenga, 1980). Table 1 summarizes the strategies for survival which we have discussed and alternative strategies for liberation specifically grounded in the principles of the Nguzo Saba to combat the difficulties faced by African American girls.

IMPLICATIONS FOR THE CLINICAL COMMUNITY

Clinicians who work with African American adolescent females in a variety of settings including schools, mental health clinics and the juvenile justice system are encouraged to realize that different strategies of resistance may be operative in the attitudes and behaviors of their clients. To empower young women and to enhance their development within the therapeutic alliance, we recommend that clinicians assess behaviors and attitudes in terms of resistance. Taking on the perspective of the client, is the client engaged in resistance as a survival strategy which ironically may be self-injurious, or can her resistance be understood as liberation oriented, whereby self-affirmation and community validation are the goal? The clinician can then identify and work with the African American adolescent client to identify resistance for survival and envision alternative strategies, or to support resistance for liberation. We provide an example of how a clinician might identify and support resistance for liberation in clinical work with an African American girl. "Carla" represents for us many black girls with whom we have spoken, read about, or whom we have known and been ourselves.

Carla is a very bright sixteen-year-old African American high school junior who dreams of going to college someday. Although Carla is well-liked by her peers, over the last year her conflicts with school personnel have steadily increased. Teachers have labelled her disruptive class behavior as overly aggressive, belligerent and "anti-social." Carla states that she is angry because her teachers are domineering and do not really care what happens to students in her large, urban school. She is referred to the school counselor who, in "relabelling" (see Pinderhughes, 1989) her behavior as

TABLE 1. Contrasting Resistance Strategies Employed by African American Girls

Resistance Strategy	
Survival/Oppression	Liberation/Empowerment
• Isolation and disconnectedness from the larger African American community.	• Unity with African people that transcends age, socio-economic status, geographic origin, and sexual orientation (Umoja).
• Self defined by others (the media, educational system) in a manner that oppresses and devalues blackness.	• Self-determination through confrontation and repudiation of oppressive attempts to demean self. New models used to make active decisions that empower and affirm self and racial identity (Kujichagulia).
• Excessive individualism and autonomy; racelessness.	• Collective work and responsibility; the self is seen in connection with the larger body of African people, sharing a common destiny (Ujima).

TABLE 1 (continued)

• "I got mine, you get yours" attitude.	• Cooperative economics advocating a sharing of resources through the convergence of the "I" and the "We" (Ujaama).
• Meaninglessness in life, immediate gratification to escape life's harsh realities, the use of "quick fixes."	• Purpose in life that benefits the self and the collective, endorses delaying gratification as a tool in resistance (Nia).
• Maintaining status quo, replicating existing models, although they may be irrelevant.	• Creativity through building new paradigms for the community, through dialogue with other resistors (Kuumba).
• Emphasis on the here and now, not looking back and not looking forward, myopic vision.	• Faith through an intergenerational perspective where knowledge of the history of Africa and other resistors and care for future generations gives meaning to struggle and continued resistance (Imani).

resistance, can help Carla to identity her sense of fury at a school system that does not have her best interests at heart. The counselor helps Carla to recognize and channel her leadership abilities to galvanize her fellow students to action, such as collectively demanding relevant and challenging course material, improved school facilities and smaller class sizes. Thus relabelling to foster healthy resistance serves three purposes: first, it aids in establishing an empathic and supportive therapeutic relationship; second, it enables the clinician to affirm behaviors and attitudes positively that had been mislabeled and misunderstood previously; and third, the relabelling process helps the client to take responsibility for negative behaviors that are self-denigrating and, through critical analysis and confrontation, begin to make changes that are self-affirming and conducive to positive psychological development.

In cultivating healthy resistance in African American adolescent females, we recommend that clinicians incorporate an Afrocentric perspective as part of the therapeutic process. In the previous example, Carla, in collaborating with other students and uniting with them to bring about effective school change, demonstrates the first principle of the Nguzo Saba – umoja, or unity (see Table 1). A wide variety of options exist for the therapist who wishes to incorporate the aforementioned Afrocentric principles into her work with African American adolescent female clients. We acknowledge that facilitating this method in therapy may pose some challenges, particularly within cross-racial therapeutic contexts. It is crucial for the clinician who works with black clients to supplement her knowledge of the convergence of race and gender issues continuously, particularly if the clinician's education and training has provided limited exposure to African American females. It should not be the client's full–responsibility to educate her therapist about the dialectics of gender and race oppression while also contending with the presenting problem at hand.

Resistance is a powerful and persistent theme in the history of African American people. We maintain that in this current hostile sociopolitical climate, African American adolescent girls are frequently engaged in resistant attitudes and behaviors. However, we believe that clear distinctions must be made between resistance for survival and resistance for liberation. We also believe that therapists can help black girls identify their engagement in resistant strategies and frame and support resistance for liberation as an alternative to the resistance for survival that can, in the long run, be so psychologically damaging. Author Toni Morrison calls the script imposed by those in power on everyone else "The Master Narrative." In adopting a posture that supports their liberation, we encourage African American adolescent females to reject "The Master Narrative" of internalized anger and self-abnegation and, in adopting an Afrocentric cultural approach to self-affirmation and community building, cultivate "a belief in self far greater than anyone's disbelief."[4]

ENDNOTES

1. See for example Gibbs chapter in Gibbs et al., (1989a) and Lee (1989) and Franklin's chapters in Jones (1989).
2. The girls represented in this article were participants in longitudinal research projects on girls' development.
3. See endnote number two.
4. We would like to thank playwright August Wilson for his generous permission to include his eloquent words here, as well as in the title of this article.

REFERENCES

Boyd-Franklin, N. (1989). *Black families in therapy: A multisystems approach.* New York: Guilford Press.

Collins, P. H. (1989). The social construction of black feminist thought. *Signs, 14*(4), 745-773.

Desmond, S., Price, J., Hallinan, C., & Smith, D. (1989). Black and white adolescents' perceptions of their weight. *Journal of Public Health, 59*(8), 353-358.

Erikson, E. (1968). *Identity, youth and crisis.* New York: W. W. Norton.

Fine, M. (1988). De-institutionalizing educational inequity: Contexts that constrict and construct the lives and minds of public school adolescents. In *School success for students at risk: Analysis and recommendations of the council of chief state school officers* (pp. 89-119). New York: Harcourt, Brace and Jovanovich.

Fordham, S. (1988). Racelessness as a factor in black students' success: Pragmatic strategy or pyrrhic victory? *Harvard Educational Review, 58*(1) February.

Fordham, S. & Ogbu, J. (1986). Black students' school success: Coping with the burden of acting white. *Urban Review, 18*, 176-206.

Franklin, A. (1989). Therapeutic interventions with black adolescents.In R. Jones (Ed.), *Black adolescents* (pp. 309-337). Berkeley, CA: Cobb and Henry Publishers.

Fulani, L. (Ed.). (1988). *The psychopathology of racism and sexism.* New York: Harrington Park Press.

Gibbs, J. T. (1989a). Black american adolescents. In J. T. Gibbs, N. Larke, & Assc. (Eds.), *Children of color: Psychological interventions with minority youth* (pp. 179-223). San Francisco: Jossey-Bass Publishers.

Gibbs, J. T. (1989b). Black adolescents and youth: An update on an endangered species. In R. Jones (Ed.), *Black adolescents* (pp. 3-27). Berkeley, CA: Cobbs and Henry, Publishers.

Gilligan, C. (1982). *In a different voice: Psychological theory and women's development.* Cambridge, MA: Harvard University Press.

hooks, b. (in press). The oppositional gaze: Black female spectators. In M. Diawara (Ed.), *Black Cinema.* New York: Rutledge Press.

Hopson, D., & Hopson, D. (1988). Implications of doll color preference among black preschool children and white preschool children. *Journal of Black Psychology, 14*(2), 57-63.

Jones, R. (Ed.). (1989). *Black adolescents.* Berkeley, CA: Cobbs and Henry, Publishers.

Karenga, M. (1980). *Kawaida Theory.* Los Angeles: Kawaida Publications.

Ladner, J. (1971). *Tomorrow's tomorrow.* New York: Doubleday.

Lee, C. (1989). Counseling black adolescents: Critical roles and functions for counseling professionals. R. Jones (Ed.) *Black adolescents* (pp. 293-308). Berkeley, CA: Cobbs and Henry, Publishers.

Luttrell, W. (1989). Working class women's ways of knowing: Effects of gender, race and class. *Sociology of Education, 62*, 33-46.

Miller, J. B. (1976). *Toward a new psychology of women.* Boston: Beacon Press.

Nobles, W. (1980). African philosophy: Foundations for black psychology. In R. Jones, (Ed.). *Black psychology* (Second Edition) (pp.23-36). New York: Harper and Row.

Okazawa-Rey, M., Robinson, T., & Ward, J. V. (1987). Black women and the politics of skin color and hair. In M. Braude (Ed.), *Women, power and therapy* (pp. 89-102). New York: The Haworth Press, Inc.

Oliver, W. (1989). Black males and social problems: Prevention through Afrocentric socialization. *Journal of Black Studies, 20*(1), 15-39.

Pinderhughes, E. (1989). *Understanding race, ethnicity and power: The key to efficary in clinical practice.* New York: The Free Press.

Ward, J. V. (1990). Racial identity formation and transformation. In C. Gilligan, N. Lyons, & T. Hanmer (Eds.), *Making connections: the relational worlds of adolescent girls at Emma Willard School* (pp. 215-232). Cambridge, MA: Harvard University Press.

Willie, C. V. (1985). *Black and white families: A study in complementarity.* Dix Hills, NY: General Hall.

Disavowing the Self in Female Adolescence

Lori Stern

INTRODUCTION

A curious phenomenon, which I am calling "disavowing the self," has been highlighted by recent studies (Brown, 1989; Gilligan, 1989; Rogers & Gilligan, 1988). Some girls, who in preadolescence demonstrate a solid sense of self, begin in adolescence to renounce and devalue their perceptions, beliefs, thoughts, and feelings. While this disavowal of self has been seen in girls who are functioning well in schools, it has also been linked to the development of psychological symptomatology, such as eating disorders and depression (Jack, 1987; Steiner-Adair, 1986). How can we, as clinicians working with girls, understand this unexpected occurrence? Bringing together psychological theory with the words of one adolescent girl who disavows herself, I will seek to explore and shed some light on this phenomenon.

Early in this century, Freud highlighted a particular problem in female adolescence by noting that girls at this age appear to undergo what he called a "fresh wave of repression" (Freud, 1905/1962, p. 86). This observation was developed by the psychoanalysts Karen Horney (1926), Helene Deutsch (1944) and Clara Thompson (1942), who further discussed the finding. In each case, these clinicians described the startling retrenchment in adolescence of a previously strong preadolescent.

Lori Stern, EdD, is a Clinical Fellow in Psychology at Harvard Medical School and Massachusetts General Hospital and Director of Research at the Boston Evening Medical Center's Mental Health Unit. She is also a psychotherapist in private practice.

> We all assume, as does Freud, that the young girl's development into womanhood is inaugurated by a sudden increase of passivity. In 1925, I expressed a view that a 'thrust of activity' precedes this increase of passivity. In my opinion, this 'thrust of activity' is the principal characteristic of prepuberty. (Deutsch, 1944, p. 5)

Horney (1926) linked this development to the feelings of dysphoria associated with taking on male-defined values and goals. A sense of inferiority comes about when a girl attempts to deviate from her own life to that of a male, and begins to measure herself by pretensions and values that are foreign to her biological nature. She cannot but feel herself inadequate (Horney, 1926).

Thompson (1942), like Horney and Deutsch, located the beginning of problems in female adolescence by observing girls shutting down. For all three theorists, this shutting down or repression was understood in the conceptual terms of female passivity and masochism posited by Freud. The literature consistently described this process as normative.

> The tendency displayed in many women to renounce their own judgement and adopt by identification the opinions of their love objects is very typical. Women are also frequently enthusiastic partisans of ideas that apparently have been given them by others . . . Even talented women are often uncertain of the value of their own ideas until they receive them from someone else whom they respect. (Deutsch, 1944, p. 131)

This particular vulnerability for girls in adolescence was viewed as normal by these theorists and understood as a consequence of penis envy and the castration complex. Although these concepts and the Freudian psychoanalytic model have been criticized for a perspective in which masculinity is the norm and the view of femininity is one of deficiency, these observations of adolescent girls remain remarkably similar to those offered by contemporary researchers of female development, who describe adolescent girls as going underground or appearing to give up their own authority

(Brown, 1989; Gilligan, 1984; Rogers & Gilligan, 1988). The work of these theorists reports an

> erosion of self-confidence in girls between the ages of 11 and 15 . . . that went beyond the usual adolescent uncertainty and questioning to indicate a deeper conflict about the validity of what they were experiencing and seeing. (Gilligan, 1984, p. 2)

This tendency to renounce and devalue one's own perceptions, beliefs, thoughts and feelings is striking in that it runs counter to currently accepted theories of adolescence. The increased self-awareness and self-reflectivity of adolescents, and the ways in which self-concept and identity are created and strengthened during this period, have inspired numerous theories and been documented in various studies (Erikson, 1958; Marcia, 1966; Offer, 1969). Yet some girls, who demonstrate a solid sense of confidence in preadolescence, begin in adolescence to repudiate their own point of view.

Why do adolescent girls disavow themselves? Although the psychological literature of this century has repeatedly documented this phenomenon, no comprehensive explanation has yet been offered. In what follows, I will discuss a girl who clearly articulates her decision to deny and ignore her own point of view. She was a participant in a three-year longitudinal study of adolescence that took place at her school (see Gilligan, Johnston & Miller, 1988). By attending to one girl's experience and bringing it together with existing psychological knowledge, steps may be taken toward a preliminary understanding of disavowing the self.

SHEILA

Sheila is a young woman enrolled at a co-educational boarding school in New England. She was interviewed each year in grades 9 through 11. In her first interview at 14, Sheila sounds very much like a "prototypical" autonomous adolescent. Integrating her capacity for self-direction with her concern for relationships, she describes herself as someone who makes decisions for herself and knows that others will still love her even if her decisions are different from theirs.

Sheila: I live by my rules because I don't look at what other people do. I look at what is best for me.

Carol: How do you decide that?

Sheila: I decide by thinking about what the consequences will be to me. . .

Carol: Have you seen yourself change since you became a teenager?

Sheila: . . . I think that before I basically believed in what my parents told me. Mom and Dad's word was all. And now I am making decisions for myself and I am capable of making these decisions. And they are going to still love me if I make decisions wrong, or make decisions different from them.

However, two years later, Sheila's decision-making takes a striking form. At 16, she describes forthrightly her decision to disavow herself, with the creation of a complex artifice, designed to protect her feelings, thoughts and beliefs from the criticism she feels certain would follow if she expressed them:

Sheila: There is always that little part jumping up in the back saying hey me, hey me, you are not worthwhile.

Carol: And why not?

Sheila: Because people have shown it. Because my relationships have proven that.

Carol: How can they show that? How do other people know?

Sheila: Other people say it has to be true because you are stupid, you don't know it yourself, you are not even worthwhile to know the truth. Other people must know it.

Carol: Do you believe that?

Sheila: In a way.

Carol: And in another way?

Sheila: In another way, I think I must be smarter because I haven't let them in.

Carol: Ah, so if you haven't let them in, then they can't know.

Sheila: I am safe, right.

Carol: But if you let them all the way in?

Sheila: Then it's not safe. Then if I do something, then I know it's me.

Carol: I see. This way you could always say they don't know the real you?

Sheila: Uh-huh. Sane, isn't it.

Carol: It is a very good hedge, but at the cost, it precludes the goal of what you have called honesty in relationships.

In this complex passage, Sheila describes a chain of events in which she responds to what she experiences as others' devaluing attitudes toward her by refusing to allow them access to that which she feels is most genuinely herself. She protects herself by agreeing with those who belittle her while knowing they are wrong because they do not truly know her. By shutting them out, she protects herself. But in defeating them, she also defeats herself, insofar as she desires "honesty in relationships."

Perhaps most unexpected is the strong sense of self that Sheila displays, even as she decides to disavow that self. She is able to articulate a clear understanding of exactly what she is doing. Throughout her three interviews she demonstrates repeated instances of this clarity in stating her convictions, while she also believes these convictions cannot be expressed. This disavowal occurs in such areas vital to relationships as deciding to drink, to have sex, and to remain in a relationship that she finds unsatisfactory. In the following passage, Sheila at 14 recounts an incident in which, against her own judgement, she engaged in excessive drinking, which she says could have resulted in the death of one friend and the arrest of another:

> A friend of mine and I and a mutual friend went out and we got really drunk, and my friend almost went into a coma because of it and that was the wrong decision . . . I think the decision was wrong for me because I was listening to what other people were telling me to do and that's just really stupid . . . It was dangerous to her life. She could have died that night. It's dangerous to him [friend who procured liquor]. He could have gone to jail. It wasn't as dangerous for me, but if he had gone to jail, Lord knows, I would have felt really bad. Or if she had died . . . It was just stupid.

Even in an intensely relational activity such as sex, Sheila is ready to ignore her own feelings and desires. She describes feeling vulnerable to agreeing to have sex with a boy, in spite of her certainty that she does not want to do so. Although she has a well–defined position in this matter, she fears that if she were to express it, she would allow herself to be convinced otherwise. She avoids this potential difficulty by not discussing her true feelings:

> When my friend came down from California, he wanted to sleep together and I didn't want to, because at that point I felt like we were drifting apart and there wasn't that much left in it. It was a hard decision because if I had said that to him, obviously what's he going to say. 'I'll be here forever, we'll always be together.' That is obviously what he is going to say. And I probably would have fallen for it.

Sheila says that she would overlook her own clearly articulated viewpoint willingly, even knowing that disappointment would follow. A year later, with a different boyfriend, she decides again not to voice her own wishes. In this case, she is certain that it is not in her best interest to continue her relationship with him, as he is several years older and involved with drugs. However, she expects that she will abandon her resolve to break up with him. She says that her preoccupation with this troubling dilemma causes her migraine headaches and makes her unable to study. Yet she fears she would upset him if she were to bring up her true feelings. In this case, she feels both that she must speak and that she cannot. Again, she describes her dilemma with startling clarity:

> It is like two people standing on a boat that they both know is sinking. I don't want to say anything to you because it will upset you and you don't want to say anything to me because it will upset you. And we are both standing here in water up to our ankles watching it rise and I don't want to say anything to you.

With this metaphor of a sinking ship, Sheila expresses her perceived helplessness in facing this dilemma. Both self and relationship are sinking quickly, and she feels as though she is at sea with no protection. The cost of either expressing herself or not expressing herself is overwhelmingly high. In the face of this problem, she tries molding herself to his wishes:

> I tried to get into his needs, doing what he wanted, and to be the person that he wanted to be with. But I am not that person, I can't be that person. Then I tried, can I give him what that person would give? I couldn't even do that. And at that point I was making myself so miserable that I figured he is not getting anything out of this, and he realizes what is going on. He has to.

In this passage, Sheila is aware of the purposelessness of what she is doing. To create an altered self for the sake of a relationship would result in destroying that relationship. To be authentic in relationship is at once too dangerous yet essential for her. She links this conflict to her experience of disappointments in relationships and of feeling vulnerable to the criticism of others. She protects herself against criticism by interacting artificially, leaving in relationships what she knows to be a mere counterfeit of herself. This strategy, designed to sustain her self-esteem in the face of attack, comes at a high cost. She does not reveal herself to anyone, and so remains out of true relationship.

Counterintuitively, Sheila shows that disavowing the self can occur hand in hand with a strong sense of self. While the self can be well articulated, it is not allowed into relationship. In an effort to protect the self, relationships become false. Thus, relationships are sacrificed in hopes of preserving the self; however, since the self depends on its relationships and vice versa, this move is an effort destined to fail. Sheila acknowledges her awareness of the futility of this strategy with her metaphor of the sinking ship.

TOWARD AN UNDERSTANDING OF DISAVOWING THE SELF

Psychological theories all point to the critical role of relationships in enhancing or inhibiting one's ability to value oneself. For girls like Sheila, the role of relationships in developing self-esteem may be particularly strong. Psychoanalytic theorists (Deutsch, 1944; Freud, 1905/1962; Horney, 1926), adolescent developmental theorists (Erikson, 1968; Marcia, 1966; Offer, 1969), and theorists of female development (Chodorow, 1974; Gilligan, 1977; Miller, 1976) all emphasize the special significance of relationship in every aspect of the girl's developing self.

However, charting the actual place of self and relationship in this development has been far more controversial for theorists, partly because of the conceptual difficulty in separating self from relationship. Some theorists emphasize the self as fundamental for relationships (e.g., Erikson, 1963) while others emphasize relationships as fundamental for the self (e.g., Kohut, 1971; Winnicott, 1960). The associated disagreement regarding the starting and ending points of development may reflect ideology as much as empiricism.

The attempt to separate self and relationship in order to clarify the interaction between them consistently presents conceptual conflicts. In one view, theorists suggest that adolescent self development proceeds by detachment from relationship (e.g., Erikson, 1963). This view places the self in opposition to relationship, which may be untenable for people in general but is considered by psychoanalytic, female developmental, and adolescent developmental theorists to be particularly inaccurate for women (e.g., Chodorow, 1974; Erikson, 1968; Freud, 1905/1962).

These theorists describe instead the primacy of relationship at all stages of women's psychological development. However, comparable difficulties are encountered by seeing the female self as totally congruent with its relationships. Viewing the self as completely able to absorb the agendas of others becomes the mirror image of seeing the self as completely outside of relationships.

Adolescent girls like Sheila may see the interplay between self and other not as a conceptual debate but as a challenging dilemma that is central to their lives. This issue has been described by theorists as a fundamental conflict throughout female psychology (Gilligan, 1977), yet recent research suggests that it is a problem that comes into particular ascendancy for girls in adolescence (Brown, 1989; Gilligan, 1984).

It is not surprising that adolescence represents a critical period for confronting this issue. Theorists of adolescence describe a time of separation, individuation, and autonomy seeking, while theorists of female development observe that the importance of strong relationship does not abate. Thus adolescent girls enter a peculiar developmental crossroads where the path to maturity would involve separation, while the path to womanhood would require connection (Stern, 1990a). The problem of disavowing the self appears directly related to this dilemma – in fact, it may even be an attempted solution (Stern, 1990b).

By disavowing the self, a girl may be attempting to avoid the choice between self and others. Denying any views that might cause conflict, she protects herself from the criticism or attack that she feels would surely follow her revelation of these views. In addition, she protects the relationship from discord that she feels could lead to a rupture.

However, this solution leads to further problems. The underlying logic is untenable: When one holds one's true views and feelings outside of a relationship, the relationship becomes unauthentic. If the relationship is false, then the self, which depends on the relationship for sustenance, also suffers. If self and relationship are inextricably intertwined, girls cannot hold out on one without diminishing the other.

IMPLICATIONS FOR THERAPY AND COUNSELING

This work raises the potential of a fundamental paradigm shift for clinicians working with adolescent girls. Until recently, theorists framed the turbulence of adolescence as a primarily male phenomenon (Marcia, 1980). However, recent research indicates that adolescence is a time of great psychological danger for girls (Petersen, 1988). A recent review of the literature cites numerous ways in which girls lose significant psychological ground during adolescence. Compared to boys, they show more depression and have poorer emotional well-being (Ebata, 1987; Rutter, 1986), exhibit more negative self appraisal (Gove & Herb, 1974; Handel & Davies, 1982), and are more likely to encounter their first psychological disturbances (Ebata, 1987). Moreover, difficulties manifested in adolescence are reported to develop often into serious adult mental illness (Rutter, 1980; Weiner & DelGaudio, 1976).

Indeed, there are strong indications that once activated, the process of disavowing the self will be sustained into adulthood. McIntosh (1984) describes problems of adult professional women in terms very similar to the disavowing of the self that I have observed in female adolescence. Among women highly accomplished in their fields, she says, it is common to feel "illegitimate, apologetic, undeserving, anxious, tenuous, out-of-place, misread, phony, uncomfortable, incompetent, dishonest, guilty" (McIntosh, 1984, p. 1). This observation suggests that disavowing the self represents a critical vulnerability in female development, with lifelong implications for a woman's psychological well-being.

The study of Sheila and other adolescent girls (Stern, 1990b) indicates that a girl's decision, conscious or unconscious, to disavow herself can exist alongside clear and direct statements of who she knows herself to be: Statements questioning her own worth coincide with statements that confirm it. In this way, girls exhibit evidence of a strong sense of self, even as they choose to disavow that self. This choice represents an active process, not properly described by terms such as "identity diffusion" or "loss of sense of self." It is an attempted solution to the problem of how to stay in connection – a solution in which the self that is known is unacknowledged.

For clinicians working with women, the recognition of adolescence as a critical period for disavowing the self poses important implications for practice. For some women, it may prove as helpful to focus on the relational disappointments of adolescence as to uncover the problematical situations of early childhood.

The greatest difficulty that this condition presents for those who work with adolescent girls is its coexistence with the appearance of well-being. Sheila could be seen as excelling in many of her pursuits: She is a successful student at a challenging preparatory school. However, her success is in goals with which she does not identify. She has never dared to examine, much less pursue, her own goals.

How can psychologists help such girls to pursue their own goals? How can these girls learn to heed their own voices? Further research is needed to develop strategies for clinicians working with girls to intervene in this process; however, an understanding of how and why girls disavow themselves is a needed first step. Therapists and counselors may reconsider their approaches to these girls if they understand disavowing the self to be not a problem of the self– for the- self can be clearly known and plainly articulated – but a problem of relationship.

REFERENCES

Brown, L. (1989). *Narratives of relationship: The development of a care orientation in girls 7 to 16.* Unpublished doctoral dissertation, Harvard University.

Chodorow, N. (1974). Family structure and feminine personality. In M. Rosaldo, & L. Lamphere (Eds.), *Women, culture, and society* (pp. 43-66). Stanford, CA: Stanford University Press.

Deutsch, H. (1944). *Psychology of women* , Vol. I. New York: Grune & Stratton.

Ebata, A. (1987). *A longitudinal study of psychological distress during early adolescence.* Unpublished doctoral dissertation, Pennsylvania State University.

Erikson, E. (1958). *Young man Luther.* New York: Norton.

Erikson, E. (1963). *Childhood and society.* New York: Norton.

Erikson, E. (1968). *Identity, youth and crisis.* New York: Norton.

Freud, S. (1905/1962). The transformations of puberty. In *Three essays on the theory of sexuality.* New York: Basic Books.

Gilligan, C. (1977). In a different voice: Women's conceptions of the self and morality. *Harvard Education Review, 47*, 481-517.

Gilligan, C. (1984). *New perspectives on female adolescent development.* Unpublished manuscript, Harvard University.

Gilligan, C. (1989). Teaching Shakespeare's sister. In C. Gilligan, N. Lyons, & T. Hanmer (Eds.), *Making connections: The relational worlds of adolescent girls at Emma Willard School.* Cambridge, MA: Harvard University Press.

Gilligan, C., Johnston, D., & Miller, B. (1988). *Moral voice, adolescent development, and secondary education: A study at the Green River School.* (Monograph No 3). Cambridge, MA: The Center for the Study of Gender, Education, and Human Development, Harvard University.

Gove, W. & Herb, T. (1974). Stress and mental illness among the young. *Social Forces, 53*, 256-265.

Horney, K. (1926). The Flight from Womanhood. *International Journal of Psychoanalysis, 7*, 324-339.

Jack, D. (1987). Silencing the self: The power of social imperatives in female depression. In R. Formanek & A. Gurian (Eds.), *Women and depression: A lifespan perspective* (pp. 161-181). New York: Springer Publishing Company.

Kandel, D. & Davies, M. (1982). Epidemiology of depressive mood in adolescents. *Archives of General Psychiatry. 39*, 1205-1212.

Kohut, H. (1971). *The analysis of the self.* New York: International Universities Press.

Marcia, J. (1966). Development and Validation of Ego Identity Status. *Journal of Personality and Social Psychology, 3*, 551-558.

Marcia, J. (1980). Identity in adolescence. In J. Adelson (Ed.), *Handbook of adolescent psychology.* New York: Wiley.

McIntosh, P. (1984). Feeling like a fraud. *Work in Progress,* No. 18. Wellesley, MA: Stone Center Working Paper Series.

Miller, J.B. (1976). *Toward a new psychology of women.* Boston: Beacon Press.

Offer, D. (1969). *The psychological world of the teenager.* New York: Basic Books.

Petersen, A. (1988). Adolescent development. *Annual Review of Psychology, 39*, 583-607.

Rogers, A. & Gilligan, C. (1988). *Translating the language of adolescent girls: Themes of moral voice and stages of ego development.* (Monograph No. 6). Cambridge, MA: The Center for the Study of Gender Education and Human Development, Harvard University.

Rutter, M. (1980). *Changing youth in a changing society: patterns of adolescent development and disorder.* Cambridge: Harvard University Press.

Rutter, M. (1986). The developmental psychopathology of depression: Issues and perspectives. In M. Rutter, C. Izzard, & P. Read (Eds.), *Depression in young people: Developmental and clinical perspectives.* New York: Guilford Press.

Steiner-Adair, C. (1986). The body politic: Normal female adolescent development and the development of eating disorders. *Journal of the American Academy of Psychoanalysis, 14*, 95-114.

Stern, L. (1990a). Conceptions of separation and connection in female adolescents. In C. Gilligan, N. Lyons, & T. Hanmer (Eds.), *Making connections: The relational worlds of adolescent girls at Emma Willard School* (pp. 73-87). Cambridge: Harvard University Press.

Stern, L. (1990b). *Disavowing the self in female adolescence. A case study analysis.* Unpublished doctoral dissertation, Harvard University.

Thompson, C. (1942). Cultural pressures in the psychology of women. *Psychiatry, 5*, 331-339.

Weiner, I. & DelGaudio, A. (1976). Psychopathology in adolescence. *Archives of General Psychiatry, 33*, 187-193.

Winnicott, D. W. (1960). *The maturational processes and the facilitating environment: Studies in the theory of emotional development.* New York: International Universities Press.

Teen Females in Minnesota: A Portrait of Quiet Disturbance

Linda Harris
Robert W. Blum
Michael Resnick

Over the past 30 years there has been a dramatic shift in the causes of mortality among young people in the United States; violence (unintentional injuries, homicides and suicides) now accounts for more than three out of every four deaths in the second decade of life. As disturbing as this observation is, when we looked more closely and explored morbidity and mortality by gender, we began to see some significant and dramatic differences. As we report here, based on the results of a large-scale study of adolescent health, adolescent males tend to be engaged in acting-out behaviors, such as fights, homicides and vandalism, while adolescent females display a picture of quiet disturbance. For girls, distress appears to turn inward. As a consequence, girls' cries for help may be harder to hear and easier to ignore.

Linda J. Harris is Project Director of the National Adolescent Health Resource Center at the Adolescent Health Program, University of Minnesota. In her spare time, she is completing her PhD in Sociology, co-anchoring a family, and as a consequence of all of the above, keeping local feminist therapists busy.

Robert William Blum, MD, PhD, MPH, is Director of the Adolescent Health Programs, University of Minnesota, and Professor and Chairperson of the Department of Pediatrics, University of Minnesota.

Michael D. Resnick, PhD, is Associate Professor of the School of Public Health, and Director of Research for the Adolescent Health Program, Department of Pediatrics. His primary interest is in adolescent health and risk behaviors, and the translation of research into social policy and programs.

Supported in part by grants #MCJ-00985 and #MCJ-273A03-01-0 Maternal and Child Health Bureau, Rockville, Maryland, and a grant from the Minnesota Women's Fund.

METHODS

The Minnesota Adolescent Health Survey was administered in the 1986-1987 school year to 36,284 youths in the seventh through twelfth grades in the state of Minnesota. The survey asked questions about students' home life, their interactions with parents and peers, school performance, levels of stress, self-esteem and body image, use of drugs, history of abuse, suicide attempts and sexual behaviors.

The demographic composition of the survey sample was comparable to the population of youth in public schools across Minnesota: 94% were white, and 6% were from ethnic or racial minority backgrounds. A third of the students surveyed lived in urban areas, a third were from rural communities, and a third lived in suburbs or small towns. Eighty percent of the students surveyed lived in two-parent households. Half of the survey respondents were female. Consequently, the results of this study reflect the general population of youth in public schools in Minnesota.

GENDER DIFFERENCES IN YOUTH RISK BEHAVIOR

When we explored the psychological differences between males and females, what emerged was a portrait of females who are far more dissatisfied with themselves than their male counterparts who are more prone to self-injurious behaviors.[1]

Body image. Females differ from males most dramatically in the area of body image and concern over their looks. "Body image" refers to the positive or negative attitude one has with respect to his or her own body and was measured by several self-report questions that asked how much pride the respondent has in his or her body, as well as their satisfaction with body weight. Girls are much more concerned about their physical appearance than are boys. Almost a third of the adolescent females (32%) express a high degree of concern about their appearance, compared to only 13% of males. A much higher proportion of the girls in this study appear to have a very negative attitude towards their bodies than the males do, and this disparity tends to increase with age. In junior high school (grades seven through nine), 30% of adolescent females report a negative body image, compared to 12% of their male counterparts. Among senior high school students (grades 10 through 12), negative body image rises to 40% among females but only to 15% among senior high males.

A "distorted" body image reflects a belief that one is overweight when one is actually of average weight for their height and frame. Based on the student's self-reported height and weight, three times as many females as males, who are of average weight for their height and age, feel that they are overweight. This preoccupation on the part of girls with how their bodies look, when coupled with a distorted body image, can lead to both chronic dieting and disordered eating. Chronic dieting is indicated by frequent or continuous patterns of eating behavior directed towards loss of weight. A respondent who indicated she had gone on a weight loss diet ten or more times in the past year, or was 'always dieting' was considered to be a chronic dieter. Chronic dieting was reported by 10% of junior high and 16% of senior high females, while only 2% of males at any grade level reported similar behaviors.

Behaviors and beliefs associated with bulimia nervosa – a particular form of disordered eating–were also reported by students who took the survey. (Questions related to anorexia nervosa, another form of disordered eating, were not asked on this survey.) Such behaviors included binging (eating large quantities in a small amount of time) and purging (vomiting, or using diuretics, laxatives or Ipecac). Almost one third of all females reported having had episodes of binge-eating followed by vomiting. Fourteen percent said they vomited purposefully at least once a month after eating. The beliefs or attitudes associated with bulimia include feelings of being out of control while eating. Based on these self-reported patterns of eating and beliefs about eating, approximately 52% of junior high school females and 65% of girls in senior high were at moderate to high risk for having or developing an eating disorder (bulimia) compared with 29% of males across all grade levels (see Figure 1).

Emotional stress and suicide. In many studies, far more adolescent females evidence symptoms of emotional stress and depression than do males (Earls, 1987; Gjinde, Block & Block, 1988; Ostrov,

TABLE 1. Adolescent Female Vulnerability by Level of Family Connectedness

	Family Connectedness* Level				
Risk Factor	Very Low	Low	Moderate	High	Overall Risk Level
High Eating Disorders Risk	6.9	3.7	2.0	1.4	3.0
High Pregnancy Risk	12.3	8.2	5.6	6.0	7.2
Negative Body Image	53.0	41.4	31.6	23.3	35.2
History of Abuse	40.7	25.8	13.8	10.1	19.7
High/Very High Emotional Stress	38.7	21.2	12.1	6.4	15.7
High Suicide Risk	13.4	3.5	1.4	1.3	3.2

*Family connectedness reflects adolescent's agreement rating of six statements such as "your parents are about you," "you get upset at home," "your family cares about your feelings," "people in your family understand you," etc.

Offer & Howard, 1989). Far more teenage girls also attempt suicide than do boys (Earls, 1987; Simons & Murphy, 1985; Wodarski & Harris, 1987). More males, however, die during their teenage years from suicide attempts than do their female counterparts because of the lethality of their attempts. Among Minnesota youth, at every grade level after the seventh, twice as many females as males reported having attempted suicide at least once. By their senior year, eighteen percent of girls reported having attempted suicide compared with nine percent of boys. For those in urban areas, the data are even more disconcerting: Nearly 23% of females reported having attempted suicide at least once. (See Figure 2.)

The gender differences for emotional stress parallel the pattern for suicidal behavior. The respondent's level of emotional stress was measured by seventeen questions which asked respondents how they felt over the last month in terms of nervousness, hopelessness, restfulness, sadness and anxiety, as well as about his or her feelings of being in control, being dissatisfied with life, etc. Those who indicated they felt high levels of most or all of these feelings were described as being at high levels of emotional stress. A higher proportion of females than males at both the junior high and senior high level manifest high levels of stress: a quarter of junior high school females (25.3%) and over a third of senior high females (36.3%), compared to 14% of junior high males, and 20% of senior high males.

Sexual behaviors. It is during adolescence when most females as well as most males start to explore their sexuality, and many begin to have sexual intercourse. While such sexual exploration may reflect normal development, it can also result in serious consequences such as unintended pregnancies or sexually-transmitted diseases. While most youth negotiate this transition to sexual activity without such dire consequences, those who do not can be affected for life. Particularly for females, an unintended pregnancy during adolescence may determine or limit later opportunities. Overall, girls report first having sexual intercourse at a later age than do males. By the time they reach 12th grade, however, there are few gender differences for either urban or rural teens: 64% of females and 61% of males have engaged in sexual intercourse (see Figure 3). Among sexually active females, unprotected intercourse or use of ineffec-

FIGURE 1. Risk for Developing Eating Disorders by Gender and Grade Level

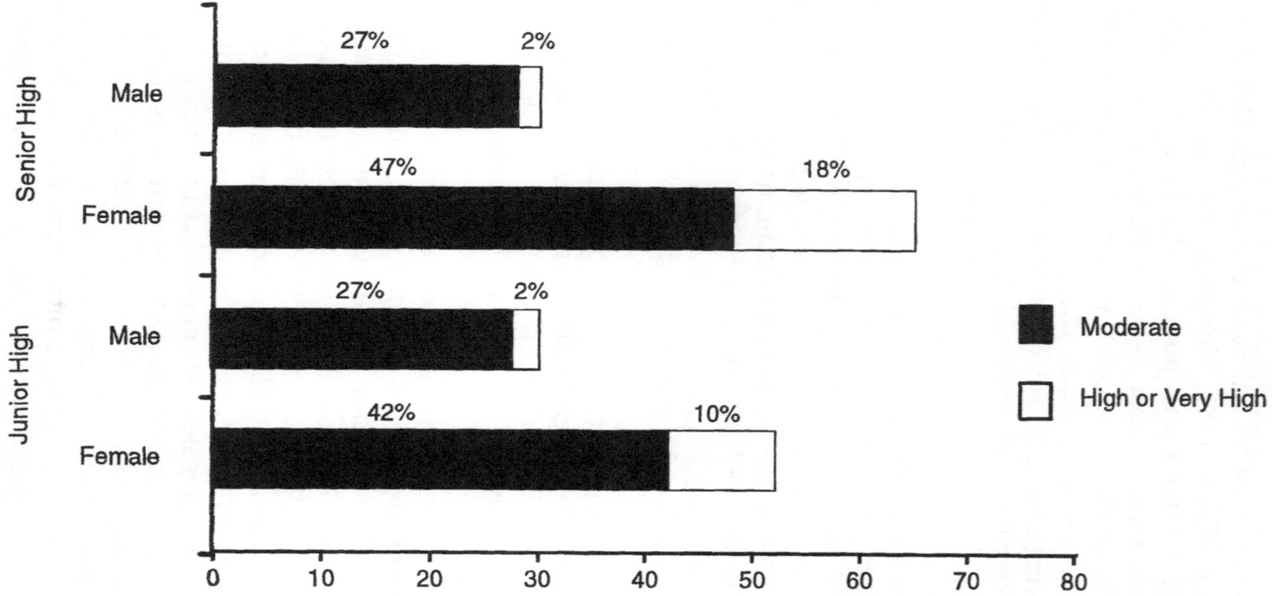

Percentage of students who are at moderate or high to very high risk for developing eating disorders.

FIGURE 2. Percentage of Suicide Attempts by Grade & Gender

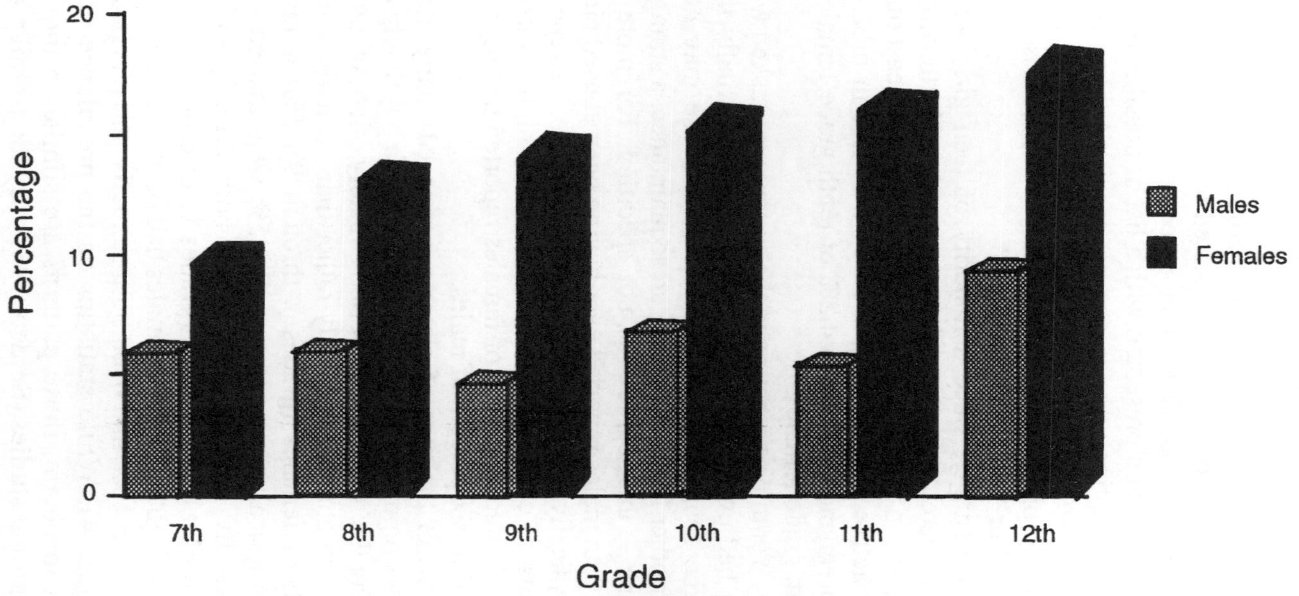

Percentage of students in grades 7 through 12 who say they have ever tried to commit suicide.

tive means of contraception remain commonplace. About three out of ten sexually active females reported using oral contraception as their primary method. Thirty-nine percent reported using no form of birth control. When presented with a list of possible reasons for not using contraception, the most frequently cited reasons included "having unexpected or unplanned sex," "didn't think of it," "didn't think pregnancy would occur," "embarrassed to get contraception," or "pregnancy desired."

Not surprisingly, since a majority of teen girls were sexually active and were not using reliable methods of birth control, a sizeable proportion reported having been pregnant at least once. Among sexually-active females in this study who live in urban areas, the rate of pregnancy rose from 4.2% of tenth grade females to 11.6% of twelfth grade females.

Abuse. Youth participating in the survey were asked whether they felt they had ever been abused physically or sexually in their lifetimes. The source or perpetrator of the abuse may have been a parent or other family member, an acquaintance, a stranger, a friend or anyone – the source was not specified. Far more adolescent females than males reported ever having been abused either sexually or physically. Five percent of junior high males reported having been abused, compared to 15% of junior high females. Among senior high students, 24% of females reported having been abused, compared to six percent of males.

In terms of the type of abuse experienced, many more females than males reported having been abused both physically and sexually. Among the males who reported a history of abuse, most reported having been abused physically rather than sexually. Among junior high school females (grades 7 through 9), 5% of females were abused physically but not sexually, 5% were abused sexually but not physically, and 5% were abused both sexually and physically. Among senior high students (grades 10 through 12), these figures increased slightly – 7% of females had been abused physically, 7% sexually, and 10% had been both sexually and physically abused (see Figure 4). While statistics on the prevalence of abuse are difficult to obtain, these patterns are similar to those found in other national studies (Seiden, 1989). By their senior year, over a quarter of the females in the study recognize and are willing to

FIGURE 3. Percent Ever Having Had Sexual Intercourse by Grade, Gender and Region

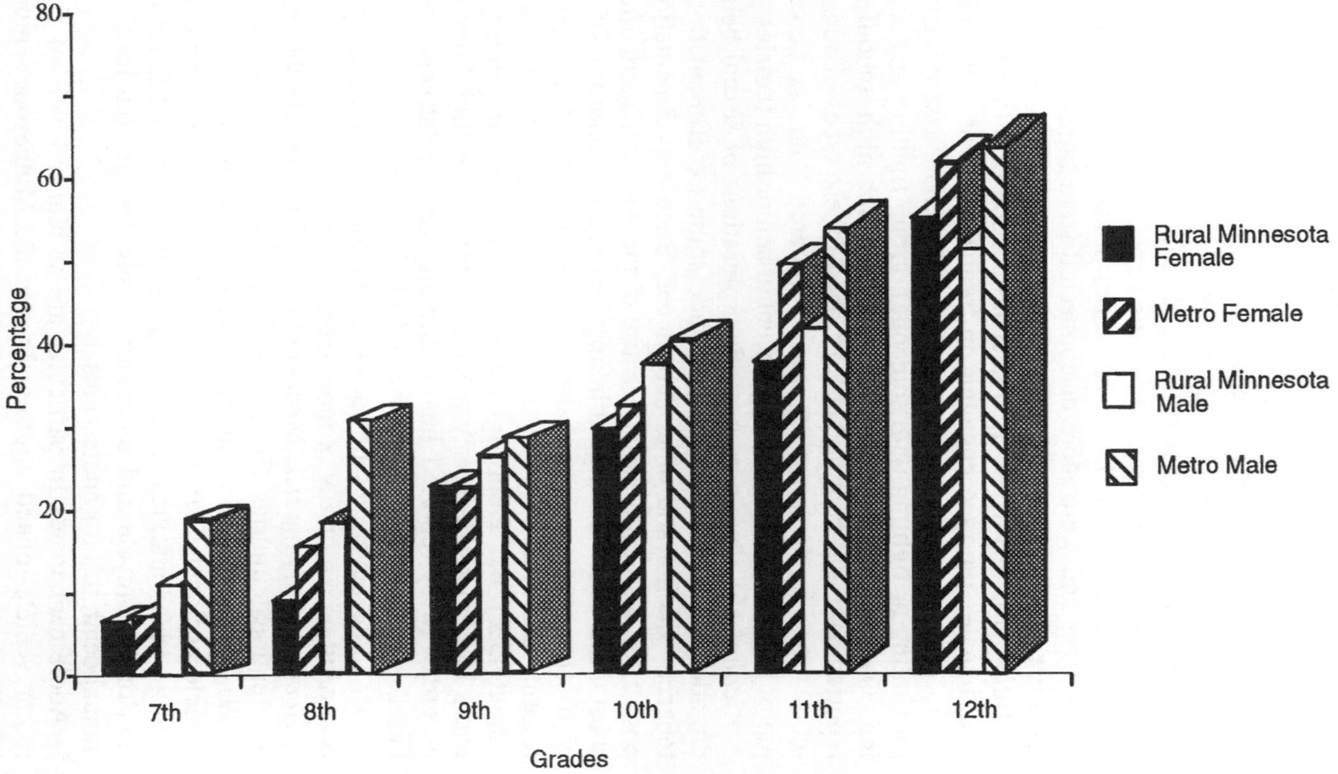

report via the survey that they have been abused in some way. Nearly three out of ten girls who were physically abused, and four out of ten girls who were sexually abused, reported they have never discussed their experience of being abused with anyone. Girls with a history of abuse also reported doing very poorly in school, were at higher risk for suicide based on current ideation and past histories of attempts and were more disconnected from family support systems than girls who had not reported a history of abuse.

Anti-social behaviors. A higher proportion of adolescent males than females reported engaging in frequent acts of anti-social behavior such as vandalism or property destruction, assaultive behavior (hitting or fighting with someone), group fighting and shoplifting. Over a tenth of both junior and senior high school males reported having committed at least one of these types of acts ten or more times in the previous year, compared with six percent of junior high females and three percent of senior high females.

Alcohol and drug use. As with explorations of sexual behavior, the adolescent years typically include some experimentation with tobacco, alcohol and other substances. Such experimentation can pose a serious health threat because of the way teenagers often use substances, such as binge drinking. An equal proportion of junior high school males and females responding to the Minnesota Adolescent Health Survey reported ever having consumed alcohol (about 45%). By senior high school, however, some gender differences had emerged. Nearly twice as many senior high boys (29%) as girls (13%) reported heavy drinking on a relatively frequent basis. Heavy drinking was defined by the researchers as drinking six or more beverages per drinking episode, with these episodes occurring on a monthly or more frequent basis.

Accidental injury risk. Most adolescent fatalities are the result of unintentional injuries (Blum, 1987; Rosen, Xiangdong & Blum, 1989). Many of these fatalities and injuries are related to motor vehicle accidents. Practices such as driving while intoxicated or riding with an intoxicated driver, failure to use seatbelts, and operation of motorcycle and recreational vehicles all contribute to the annual death toll for adolescents.

Adolescent males in particular are at higher levels of risk for motor vehicle-related injuries. Among the Minnesota senior high school youth surveyed, more males (27%) than females (21%) reported ever having driven after drinking. About equal proportions of males and females (28%) reported often or sometimes riding with someone who has consumed alcohol or other drugs. Females were much more likely to report using seatbelts regularly than males (47% versus 35%). Males were also more likely to have reported riding motorcycles or recreational vehicles monthly or more often than females (29% of males, compared to 13% of females). These are some of the factors which place males at greater risk for accidental injury than females.

SUMMARY OF GENDER DIFFERENCES

What emerges is a portrait of adolescent girls in significant psychological distress. Girls appear to act out that distress in self-directed, quietly disturbed behaviors. Compared with boys the same age, more girls report having a distorted body image and being at high risk for eating disorders or chronic dieting. Proportionately more adolescent females are at higher levels of emotional stress and are more likely to make suicide attempts than boys. Adolescent females are also more likely to report having been sexually or physically abused, and a majority of these females reported not having discussed this experience with anyone else or having sought help.

These findings mirror many other studies of gender differences among adolescents. From clinic populations, school-based populations and general populations, females have been found to tend towards internalized expressions of distress such as those noted above, while males have tended towards externalized expressions of distress, such as delinquent anti-social behaviors, aggression, substance abuse, and extreme risk-taking (Earls, 1987; Garber, 1984; Gjinde, Block & Block, 1988; Harlow, Newcomb & Bentler, 1986; Ostrov et al., 1989; Seiden, 1989; The Minnesota Women's Fund, 1990).

Previous researchers have suggested that these differences in males and females expressions of distress reflect differences in socialization from a very young age. What is not understood is the relationship between depression or emotional stress and acting out behaviors. Which comes first? Does emotional stress "cause" some adolescents to act out or does acting out cause some adolescents to become depressed? Does acting out behavior mask some forms of stress or depression among adolescents? Some researchers have suggested that for males in particular, the acting out behaviors receive attention, and consequently a label (conduct disturbance), while an underlying emotional problem is often unrecognized (Garber, 1984; Gjinde et al., 1988).

This characterization of adolescent females as being more prone to internalization of stress and adolescent males as being more prone to externalized expressions may be an oversimplification of gender stereotypes. We found that, in fact, these two modes of coping crosscut gender lines to a certain extent – some females engage in acting out behaviors, and some males also appear to direct their distress internally. Nor are these manifestations mutually exclusive – a certain proportion of both males and females engage in acting out behaviors and also exhibit self-directed destructive behaviors. The association between these two modes of expression of distress is probably complex. Further longitudinal research on general populations is needed to delineate the link between these expressions of distress. For mental health professionals, the coexistence of acting out and quietly disturbed behaviors should be explored.

SOCIAL FACTORS AND GENDER DIFFERENCES

As noted, the propensity either to act out or to turn one's distress inward seems to be gender-related: Boys are more likely to act out, and girls are more likely to be quietly disturbed. However, the role of other factors in these gender differences is less well understood. The ways in which heredity, school environment, family environment or other factors interact with gender to predispose adolescents to problems or to particular modes of expression of psychological distress has been largely unexplored.

In other studies, family factors have been shown to have a strong effect on young children's behavior (Earls, 1987). In the Minnesota study, the quality of family relationships is of primary importance in emotional distress among both boys and girls. A discriminant analysis was conducted on the Minnesota data to identify factors which predicted an absence of quietly disturbed behaviors for males and females. This approach provides clues to the social or family context factors which may protect adolescents from developing these internally-directed negative behaviors. The strongest predictor of an absence of quietly disturbed behaviors for both males and females was a strong feeling on the part of the adolescent of family connectedness. This predictor represents the degree to which the adolescent feels connected with his or her family and feels their family cares about them (The Adolescent Health Program, 1989). Among females in particular, the factors which were most strongly predictive of quietly disturbed behaviors included poor levels of family connectedness, followed by poor school performance, high levels of family stress, low levels of religiosity and older age levels. Among males, the strongest predictors of quietly disturbed behaviors were low levels of connectedness with family, followed by poor performance in school, high levels of family stress and low levels of willingness to go to peers for help with psychosocial types of problems. The similarities between the genders are much stronger than the dissimilarities – a feeling of connection with and care from family may be an important "protectant factor" for both adolescent males and females in preventing internalized distress.

Some studies have suggested that family relationships affect boys and girls differently in determining whether or how they act out or turn distress inward. For instance, several studies have shown that a family environment of marital discord and abuse is associated with more behavior problems among boys than girls (Earls, 1987). Some researchers have shown that for girls, their relationship with their parents, and with their mother in particular, has been found to have a strong preventative impact on some forms of psychopathology. Adolescent girls who report having positive relationships with their mothers have demonstrated lower levels of suicide risk (Triolo, McKenry, Tishler & Blyth, 1984), less frequent depressive forms of psychopathology (Earls, 1987), less disordered eating and more positive body images (Attie & Brooks-Gunn, in press). Some researchers suggest that a strong relationship between girls and their mothers can serve as a buffer for family or other forms of stress – a buffer which may be less available to, or at least be less effective, for boys.

Among girls in the Minnesota study who experienced lower levels of family connectedness, a very high proportion evidence quietly disturbed behaviors, such as high levels of emotional stress, negative body image, disordered patterns of eating, suicide attempts and pregnancy risk (see Table 1). In this study, the stronger the connection the teenage girl felt with her family, the less likely she was to engage in behaviors which signal psychological distress. There are factors other than family connectedness that place girls at risk, but the most powerful predictor is the quality of the relationship a girl has with her family.

CONCLUSION

This study suggests powerfully that significant numbers of adolescent girls may be psychologically distressed. However, their cry is likely to be turned inward and thus muffled. It may be more difficult to detect problems of this nature; suicidal tendencies, disordered patterns of eating and emotional stress do not often call attention to themselves until the damage is severe. This study has also reiterated the findings of other studies that a strong feeling of connectedness with parents and family emerged as the most important factor for protecting adolescent females from developing these quietly disturbed behaviors. Unfortunately, we cannot legislate strong family connections. Even under the most optimal circumstances, all children will not be nurtured in caring family environments. Other research has suggested that in lieu of such family support, a relationship with one other adult, one individual who is emotionally connected to the adolescent, increases an adolescent girl's likelihood of weathering the stress she faces in adolescence and of experiencing fewer negative life consequences (Garmezy, 1987).

This finding is of particular interest to therapists who work with adolescents. It is a sense of connection, and of being cared about by

FIGURE 4. Percent of Adolescent Girls Ever Abused by Type of Abuse and Grade

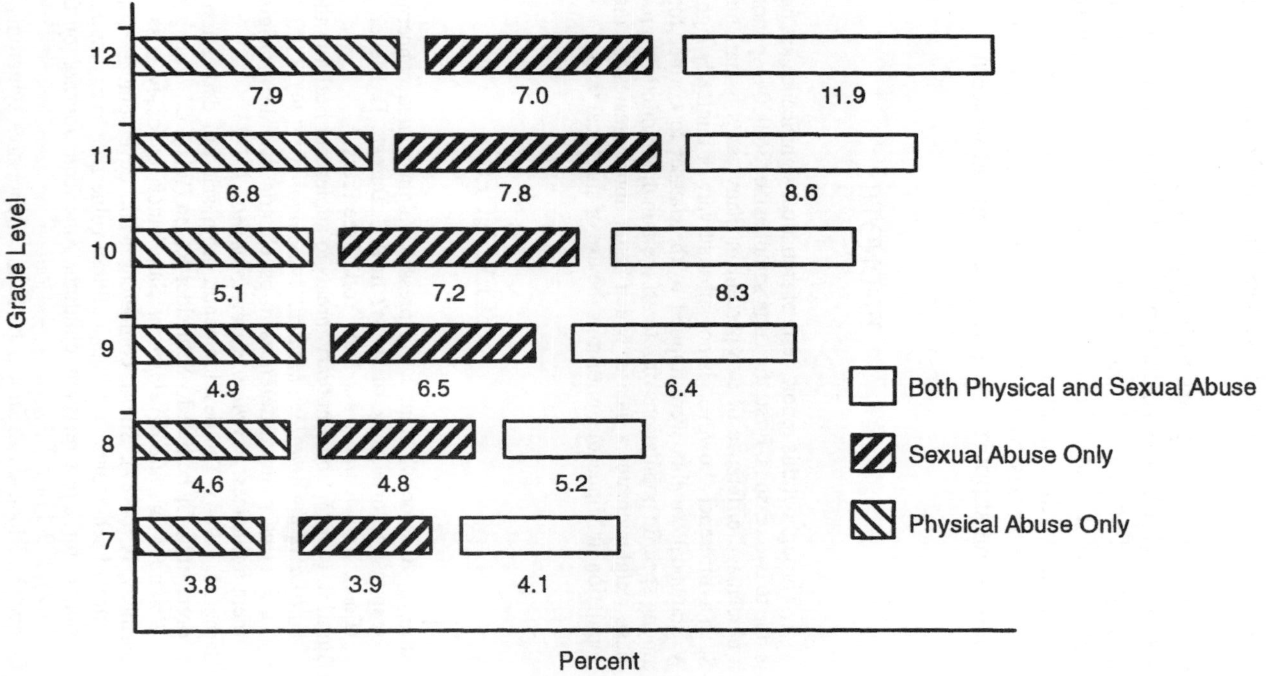

an adult, which appears to help provide resilience to psychological stresses which often accompany adolescence for females. Therapists can help fulfill that need either by trying to be that caring person for the adolescent or by helping that young person to find someone–with whom they can build such connections through making referrals to programs or services which can provide that one-on-one support and guidance to an adolescent.

ENDNOTE

1. Throughout this report, tests of statistical significance are not reported. This is due to two reasons. First, the large sample size (36,000 respondents) means that a percentage difference of two percent in many cases is statistically significant. Such a difference, however, is not substantively or clinically significant. Secondly, statistical weights were applied to the dataset to correct for over-sampling among specific populations of interest (certain urban minority groups). The use of these weights creates a dataset which better approximates the distribution of the population in Minnesota, but limits the use of statistical tests.

REFERENCES

Attie, I., & Brooks-Gunn, J. (in press). Weight-related concerns in women: A response to or a cause of stress? In R.C. Barnett, L. Biener, & G.K. Baruch (Eds.), *Women and stress.* New York: Free Press.

Blum, R. (1987). Contemporary threats to adolescent health in the United States. *Journal of the American Medical Association. 257*(24), 3390-3395.

Earls, F. (1987). Sex differences in psychiatric disorders: Origins and development influences. *Psychiatric Developments. 1*, 1-23.

Garber, J. (1984). The developmental progression of depression in female children. In D. Cichetti & K. Schneider-Rosen (Eds.), *Children's depression: New directions for child development.* San Francisco: Jossey-Bass.

Garmezy, N. (1987). Stress, competence, and development: Continuities in the study of schizophrenic adults, children vulnerable to psychopathology, and the search for stress-resistant children. *American Journal of Orthopsychiatry. 57*(2), 159-174.

Gjinde, P., Block, J., & Block, J. (1988). Depressive symptoms and personality during late adolescence: Gender differences in the externalization-internalization of symptom expression. *Journal of Abnormal Psychology. 97*(4), 475-486.

Harlow, L., Newcomb, M., & Bentler, P.M. (1986). Depression, self-derogation,

substance use, and suicide ideation: Lack of purpose in life as a motivational factor. *Journal of Clinical Psychology. 42*(1), 5-21.
Ostrov, E., Offer, D., & Howard K. (1989). Gender differences in adolescent symptomology: A normative study. *Journal for the American Academy of Childhood and Adolescent Psychiatry. 28*(3), 394-398.
Rosen, D., Xiangdong, M., & Blum, R. (1990). Adolescent health: Current trends and critical issues. *Adolescent Medicine. 1*(1), 15-31.
Seiden, A. (1989) Psychological issues affecting women throughout the life cycle. *Psychiatric Clinics of North America. 12*(1), 1-24.
Simons, R., & Murphy, P. I. (1985). Sex differences in the causes of adolescent suicide ideation. *Journal of Youth and Adolescence. 14*(5), 423-434.
The Minnesota Women's Fund (1990). *Reflections of risk: Growing up female in Minnesota, a report on the health and well-being of adolescent girls in Minnesota.* Minneapolis, MN: Author.
The Adolescent Health Program (1989). *The social health of adolescent women in Minnesota: Patterns of risk behaviors and resiliency.* Minneapolis, MN: Author.
Triolo, S., McKenry, P., Tishler, C. & Blyth, D. (1984). Social and psychological discriminants of adolescent suicide: Age and sex differences. *Journal of Early Adolescence. 4*(3), 239-251.
Wodarski, J., & Harris, P. (1987). Adolescent suicide: A review of influences and the means for prevention. *Social Work. 6*, 477-484.

SECTION III: THE CENTRALITY OF RELATIONSHIPS

Raising a Resister

Beverly Jean Smith

Throughout my reading of psychological literature and research on women, the printed word runs counter to my experiences. Ideas and concepts ring true to the larger knowledge I have of women in general and white, middle-class women in particular. This is understandable, since in my experience, individuals write out of and from what they know, feel, and live. Raised as a resister, I am able to question these paradigms. I see spaces that need filling, so that a more complete picture of women's development emerges.

This essay gives me a chance to enter a written discourse about women's experience. I speak only for myself within my family, community and school contexts, though I know that other African American women and women from different backgrounds share some of what I say. When I read the psychological literature about mother-daughter relationships, mostly what strikes me is daughters' pain, anger, hate, rejection, fear and struggle to find self. Perhaps

Beverly Jean Smith is a doctoral student in Teaching, Curriculum and Learning Environments at the Harvard Graduate School of Education. She is currently the chairperson of the *Harvard Educational Review.* A published poet, she is writing a book about her Aunt Hilda's life.

these relationships drain some adolescent girls of the energy necessary to resist others' definitional norms. This way of speaking about the mother-daughter relationship runs counter to my experience. For the first ten years of my life, when my mother was alive, she and I related in what I experienced as healthy and healing ways.

She believed in me and recognized me as an individual. Two moments flash through my mind of her backing up my voice when teachers refused or just could not hear me. I remember a time when, in kindergarten, I kept telling my teacher I was not sleepy. She kept fussing at me, because I did not take naps. Eventually I told my mother. She came to my kindergarten class and asked the teacher if I got on the cot. "Yes." Did I disturb others? "No." Was I quiet? "Yes." Then she said that was all that could be asked of me. I could not be forced to nap. In fact, even at home I did not take naps, although my sister did. My mother lost a half a day's pay. She came to school again when I was in sixth grade, because a teacher kept calling me a liar. I had been questioned by this teacher several times about a fight that had occurred away from the school grounds. She was not my classroom teacher. I reported this questioning to my mother. She always told us to tell the truth and that anything could be dealt with. My sister and I owned up to all of our actions, good or bad, and faced the music. She assured the teacher that my version of the story was the truth as I knew it. Furthermore, she did not appreciate the teacher calling me a liar and to quit doing so, since I had explained to her several times that I had told the truth about the incident.

CONNECTEDNESS AND INDEPENDENCE

My first five years of living would have most social scientists today label me "poor" and "disadvantaged." Even then, I was probably living in poverty by white societal standards: living in two rooms, sharing a communal toilet and heating water to take baths in a tin tub. I was never fazed by these conditions, because I never felt poor, which is not so uncommon. Throughout my adult life, many acquaintances have echoed similar circumstances and sentiments.

In May of the same year that my mother came to school, she died in childbirth, after giving birth to a stillborn child. I was ten, and my sister Donna was twelve. My mother was one of ten children, and my sister and I were close to her people. These relationships provided a foundation that helped keep me centered. My sister Donna and I spent the summer of 1960 in California with my mother's family. They had moved in the summer of 1959. After a series of discussions involving my Aunties, my father, and my sister and me, the two of us ended up twenty miles from St. Louis, Missouri in St. Charles. The layout of the city was mostly unfamiliar, but the neighborhood we knew. After all, nearly every Sunday early in my life, my sister and I had visited my grandmother's house and spent several weeks there every summer among family. Here my sister and I lived with my first cousin Phyllis, who was twenty-one and married with a sixteen-month-old daughter. She and her family had moved from their tiny apartment in St. Louis into Grandma's house in St. Charles in 1959.

Soon after the death of my mother, my father and I sat in the main office of Benton Elementary School, my new school, waiting to see the counselor so that I could be registered. Even though I had completed half of the sixth grade before my mother died, the counselor said I would have to repeat the whole grade. My father asked my opinion. I said, "I should be allowed to go to the seventh grade. I was a good student and had good grades." Since I had just turned eleven, the counselor said I was too young for seventh grade. He stressed that I had already missed the first three weeks of the school year. I held my ground. I wanted to be in seventh grade. If I did not do well, then they could put me back in sixth. My father agreed. The counselor told me that someone would take me to the sixth grade classroom. I protested, but when my father told me to go, I left.

The whiteness struck me as I entered the room. My schools had been full of black people: the principal, teachers and classmates. My eyes locked with the only other black student; we smiled. I knew Linda Brown from visiting my relatives year after year. I remember nothing else about this room, the teacher, or the students, only the relief that rushed over me an hour later, when someone appeared at the door and led me back to the office. To support my claim that I was a good student who could handle the seventh grade, my father had driven to St. Louis and returned with all of my report cards. My father drove me to the junior high, so I could register again. The counselor there repeated my proposition to me: If I did not do well, I would be placed in sixth grade. Over the next three weeks he called me into his office weekly to inquire if I was having any difficulties with the schoolwork. Each week I echoed the same response: "I'm doing fine and the work isn't too hard." He assured me that I could be honest about any of these difficulties, since going back to sixth grade was not a bad thing. According to whom, I thought. I decided then and there that I would do well for my mother, my family, and the black people I had left at Marshall Elementary School in St. Louis. They sustained me in these predominantly white surroundings. Their collective voices would rise inside my head or be conjured up by me.

Of course, I had seen white people before. They owned or worked in a myriad of small businesses located on the street level of most buildings in my old neighborhood. They formed a backdrop. Children jumped, skipped and walked past their windows without them affecting our lives. Excluding Leonard and Barbara, the two youngest children of the white family who lived on the block, white people were outside of "my world." We did not talk or think about them one way or the other. In my new school, as situations arose or confronted me, the voices in my head, and I engaged in what black people know as "call and response.

VOICE: THE INTERPLAY OF CALL AND RESPONSE

As an African American, I grew up within a particular cultural context that values voice. African American culture demands that individual voices be connected to the whole and not just to go solo and fly off somewhere. In the neighborhoods where I was growing up, I would often see a group of young males clustered on a corner or somebody's steps. One starts a beat, the others chime in without explicitly being asked. They have responded to the indirect call of the male who began the beat. In 1990, "a rap" will probably emerge with one male giving his verse, then fading back into the beat as another voice surfaces. A group of my female friends and I meet. A conversation begins. Before we know it, all of us are speaking at the same time on the subject that has been raised by someone. Somehow, one voice gets the lead, while the rest of us become the background music. Eventually, another voice rises to displace the previous lead voice that joins us in the background. In New Orleans, Teish calls this act gumbayaya. Attend a B.B. King or Anita Baker or Public Enemy concert and notice that the audience talks to – the performer. But nowhere is call and response stronger than in the church. On any Sunday, a conversation goes on between the preacher and his congregation. He does not simply deliver the sermon but converses with "the church." He "calls" and God has "called him." A connectedness exists for African Americans between the individual and those around her or him, in all of these scenes. From birth, I feel I have understood the triadic concept of the individual, the family, the universe.

TENDING VOICE

This triad shaped my psyche. Although I was raised by my two parents until my mother's death, I felt always that I was of a larger collective community of aunts, uncles, grandmothers, cousins, and family friends. In contrast to the ways that relationships between women in families are portrayed, I saw relationships between the women in my mother's family as anything but pathological; my mother, aunts and grandmother had a "positive connection, interdependence and mutual exchange" (Herman and Lewis, 1986, p. 160). My mother visited her family every weekend after she left home. She would take the train from St. Louis, Missouri to Augusta and be picked up in town. After she got married, we visited my grandmother every weekend. Aunt Ruth lived next door to grandma, and Aunt Bertha lived one block away from them. When grandma decided to move to California, they went too – all but Aunt Hilda, who stayed in the country and tended gardens, flower and vegetable.

ANCESTRY: THE WOMEN'S CHORUS

> Do historical, cultural, and psychoanalytic assumptions about development and maturity correspond to our own experiences?
>
> (Hirsch, 1989, p. 23)

I, girlchild in a working-class, African American family; I, the great granddaughter of Maude White who birthed one child, my grandmother, say no. Annie Hamm, my grandma, bore ten children, the first four were girls, and the last six were boys. Girl one birthed no children. Girl two birthed one child, a daughter. Girl three, my mother, birthed two daughters and died giving birth to her first son. Girl four birthed one daughter then one son. My maternal lineage illustrates that these women birthed women first. How did this pattern shape the experiences and mindset of women in my family?

My great-grandmother left my grandmother to be raised by her uncles. Her parting advice to her daughter was "don't have a lot of children." Clearly grandma did not listen. I suppose her mother meant it would tie grandma down. No such luck. With five children and no money, grandma packed them up and left grandpa when she thought he was messing around with another woman. Aunt Hilda told me that after they lived six months with grandma's twin uncles, John and Robert, grandpa came, professed his innocence and begged grandma to come back home. She did.

For my aunts and my mom, being the first four children born in a rural setting placed a lot of responsibility on them. They did gardening, housework and childrearing. They were strong-willed, independent and fiercely loyal to one another. Because they were black, they were denied the right to attend the town's white high school. The three oldest daughters graduated from elementary school together and had to move approximately fifteen miles from home to get a high school education. There they had access to the schoolbus that carried them another 35 miles (one way) to the nearest black high school located in St. Charles, Missouri. Their new male classmates acknowledged their beauty. They remarked, "mmmmm, look at those Ham girls, they look good enough to eat." To support their retort that their last name was not spelled like the meat, they changed the spelling of their last name, against my grandfather's protest, from H-a-m to H-a-m-m. All of these women before me defined their own existence against the odds. Born poor into a racist society, this larger society negated their existence, chipped away at their humanity. They were not framed within the picture that came to be scrutinized and redrawn within cultural, historical and psychoanalytic analysis. Neither was I. They and I lived in the borders.

The common understanding of women's psychological state as rooted in her powerless existence as homemaker and childrearer, or a pedestal queen, carries little weight within my family. Although the women in my family fall into the first two categories; except for my Aunt Hilda, they all worked outside of the home. In the black community I grew up in, being a mother held status, so whether women worked or did not work, if they were mothers, they were still valued. Women's work contributed to the well-being of the family unit. Their checks were not extras but necessities. In my family, all of the women handle the bills, even my Aunt Hilda who never worked outside of the home:

> *My thing to do was get the bills: get the bills figured out, read the meter so really it was my thing to keep the books whatever it was. A lot of women don't know what to do when her husband dies, like I did, cuz he don't tell her nothin and he don't want her to find out nothin!*

HOPE CHESTS AND PRINCE CHARMING

Herman and Lewis's (1986) analysis of Cinderella, Snow White, and Sleeping Beauty made me slowly shake me head in disagreement when I thought about my community:

> The resolution of the fairy tales, in which the daughter-heroine is lifted onto the prince's horse, represents not merely sexual fulfillment, but escape from the degraded female condition. Each girl is encouraged in the fantasy that an exception will be made for her; that as a princess, she will be chosen by a man to be elevated above the common drudgery of feminine existence, the drudgery to which she sees her mother consigned. (p. 152)

Princess was not a term bestowed upon the young girls in my family. The women may have reigned but not as queens sitting on pedestals. Entitlement escaped them, even "lady." "Woman" was the term of the day. It was their acts that empowered Grandmothers and Aunts. These black women were the forerunners of what later white feminists wanted to become: independent, working, jugglers of self and family.

When I entered St. Charles High School, I was often searching "the white terrain" for some glimmer of my social reality, something that reflected my world even if in just a shard of light. For instance, several of my white girlfriends commented that on their upcoming birthdays, they would be receiving two gifts: one for them, and one for their "hope chests." I queried, "What's a hope chest?" Puzzled faces and voices responded. "You don't have a hope chest?" "No, what is it?" "Well," they chimed, "it's for when you get married." Married, I'm only thirteen. Even though I had a boyfriend who was three years my senior, I was hardly thinking about marriage. They educated me about the need to purchase china, crystal and linens, so as a new bride I would already have something. I laughed, because I found it strange. Why spend money hoping when people give newlyweds gifts? "Besides," I said, "What if you don't get married?" At my last remark, they laughed and assured me they would. Perhaps embedded in their reply was their hope for a Prince Charming. The voices of my aunts spoke to me. As daughters and nieces, we, like most of my black female peers were told, "Be able to take care of yourself. Always have your own money."

No Prince Charmings would be coming on white horses. In America the concept of a "powerful black male" is an oxymoron. Not today, tomorrow or next week could we black daughters "rely on powerful men for [our] salvation" (Herman and Lewis, 1986, p. 152). Even as a fantasy, these tales were and are too farfetched against the realities of black life. Unlike the white male, the black male cannot elevate their women nor protect them. How can black men rescue black women when they cannot save themselves? Beginning in slavery, black men could not keep black women from being raped by the master. Yet the white man hung many black men or boys for just looking at their white women. Emmet Till, a fourteen-year-old boy from Chicago, was killed in the 1960's because in fun he called a white lady "baby." Black men were denied so-called status jobs and were relegated to chauffeur, shoeshine boy, train porter, or other blue collar work. White males held them in "check" or withheld the check. Since money creates a type of power, menial pay for blacks maintained white male status. The work of black men was certainly undervalued.

Both the black man and the black woman "slaved" and endured indignities within the larger society. These realities contributed to equal monetary status within male-female relationships. My aunts, mother and grandmothers did not see themselves as less than anyone. They would tell us children: "You are not better than anyone but as good as, and six feet of ground makes everybody the same size in the end." My white girlfriends asked me questions about my relationship with Robert, my boyfriend, that I found puzzling. A varsity athlete, many females, both white and black, saw him as being "fine." "Don't you want him to walk you to all of your classes? Don't you get upset when you see girls talking to him?" "No, I don't." I already knew from being in my family and my black community that women or men left one another, no matter how much time they spent together in public or in private. Also I heard black women speak these words: "Bein with somebody don't mean you own 'em." A variation served as a warning: "Don't make the mistake of actin' like you own me cuz we gave up slavery a long time ago." I responded to my white girlfriends' queries that Robert and I knew we went together and that's what mattered. Besides, he was the one who had asked me to go with him. I didn't make him do that, and I couldn't make him stay.

The realities I witnessed in my community informed the voice I shared with black people in my life. I felt no need to take on the views or ways of my white girlfriends. Their most disconcerted moment came in seventh grade, when they discovered I did not wear a bra. I didn't wear one, because I didn't need one. "But you should be wearing a training bra (something else I had never heard of), so when they grow, they won't sag." I appreciated their concern but didn't believe I'd be saggin' with or without a bra, and I continued to go braless. Another junior high incident comes to mind: me in seventh grade, determined to get out of taking the eighth grade home economics requirement. Mrs. Cereno drove me crazy, as did her projects. Sewing wasn't so bad, but everybody had to make the same pattern out of solid fabric. She permitted us to have one, two or no pockets, and one row of bric-brac above the required three-inch hem. Such conformity I could live without. I expressed my sentiments in a more appropriate manner but with no luck. Adding the ultimate insult, she made us all wear them to school on the same day and announced it over the loudspeaker system. I told her I didn't want to wear my skirt to school. She told me that was not my decision to make but hers, and it affected my grade. I wore it, knowing I would not sew another stitch for her when I got to eighth grade. Cooking proved just as trying. She required us to sample every kitchen's finished meal. When we made breakfast, I wouldn't sample eggs or french toast. Mrs. Cereno instructed me to do so. I told her politely that I didn't eat eggs or any food in which I could taste eggs. She reminded me of the rule. I repeated, "I couldn't" and clarified that eating eggs or french toast would make me sick. She marked my grade down, because I was being uncooperative. That was the last straw! I read the course catalog and made an appointment with my counselor. Since creative writing was listed as a fine art, as was home economics, I wanted to substitute it for the half-year home economics requirement. He said that ninth graders usually took that course. I observed that no restrictions were listed, and that the requirement stipulated that I needed one fine art credit to graduate, not two semesters of home economics. Reluctantly he allowed me to take creative writing. I floated out of his office.

"Speak your mind. Do what needs doin'. Be yourself. You gotta live your life for yourself." These messages enabled me to speak up. I was raised as a resister. These sayings were spoken to me and reflect my freedom and comfort to be me. If I believed I was being mistreated or if I had something to say, I was to say it. Respecting other people and accepting them for who they were, not by title, went along with speaking up. Surrounded by a large group of women: family, friends, and neighbors, I have always felt connected while acting alone.

HARMONIZING: CHORDS FOR RESISTANCE

When I am born, I cannot speak but a sound comes forth. Some call it a cry. I do not feel it as such. It is my voice branding my existence on the world. How could anyone else announce me but me? From this first moment I am whole, not a "part of" others, though I am certainly "of" them. My Aunts have different personalities, temperaments and affinities, but when it comes to us nieces, they have always been the same. "crazy" about us in sane ways. My sister says it well:

> *Growing up we didn't have to go through a lot of questioning and answering. We didn't have to ask a lot of questions, but if we asked they answered us. People didn't talk down to us. They answered us in an adult way. If they felt it wasn't any of our business, they just told us and went on doing what had to be done. Whatever we did we did. We didn't have to prove ourselves everyday, and we didn't have to have our success be reinforced. We didn't have to seek approval. I mean graduating from high school and finishing college was just another day. Even birthdays we never really celebrated, which would probably make a lot of insecurity in other people, but it didn't in us.*

Our Aunties' love for us radiates and embraces us. We know they are always in our corner. This has a healing effect, becomes an antidote for whatever obstacles we have to hurdle or hurl ourselves over. We nieces are never alone. The Aunties are not Angels-in-the-house (Woolf, 1944/1921) who try to silence us. Often they say: *"You betta learn to open up your mouth and speak for yourself."* They have always been concerned that our spirit not be broken. They would say: *"Stand up for yourself. Don't go around here poutin'. Say somethin' to somebody. We can't help if we don't know. Don't let nobody mistreat you."* We understand that includes them as well. When we were children, they would discipline us. Then and now, they disagree with some of the choices we make; still we are valued. They raise us still. We feel tied to them but not bound. They make it clear that although we are nieces, we are also Donna and Beverly. Our roles as nieces and aunties are only one aspect of each of us. We see the Aunties as real people. Aunties is a title, not the royal "we" but the collective we as thee.

Donna, my sister, says: *"I think a lot of things in me come from Aunt Hilda, like my inner calmness. I think it's collectedness (not calmness), because they made us feel secure and we didn't have to compete."* When my sister says this, I am relieved. During the first sessions of a women's psychology class, I remembered making the statement that growing up I never worried about being rejected. Nor did I feel as if I was in a power struggle with my aunts. "So to explain my ability to persist and resist, I call upon the voices of my sister and my Aunt Hilda. In telling of my psychological development, I have to connect my story to others. Throughout this paper, my voice surfaces then fades, as one of their voices comes forth. A connection with the whole family frames all of these voices. This relationship and interaction between me and the whole is a reflection of what keeps me from being silenced and keeps me above ground.

I am a daughter speaking about mothering. Aunts commit to this act of nurturing, of being connected, an act of becoming. They often speak these words: *"Havin' babies is easy, raisin' them is hard."* Tending the roots is key. Tiller and soil. Hilda and me. Great Grandma Maude, Grandma Annie, Aunt Bertha, Aunt Ruth, Momma, Donna and me. We go back to the same place, the same beginning, the countryside. Inside ourselves this place is planted. I am "of" these women and of this place. From the earliest age my mother sowed the seed of truth in me: "Never lie to me or yourself, if we know the truth we can deal with anything." Mothering and daughtering are my family's acts of faith and possibilities. A child is born. The cycle continues. Rooted and connected, I am a resister. I entered the world with a voice, and all of these women have helped me sing.

REFERENCES

Herman, J. L. & Lewis, H. B. (1986). Anger in the mother-daughter relationship. In T. Bernay & D. W. Cantor (Eds.), The psychology of today's woman: New psychoanalytic visions. Cambridge, MA: Harvard University Press.

Hirsch, M. (1989). The mother-daughter plot: Narrative, psychoanalysis, feminism. Bloomington: Indiana University Press.

Woolf, V. (1944/1921). Professions for women. In V. Woolf, A haunted house and other stories. New York: Harcourt, Brace and World.

Two-Part Inventions: Knowing What We Know

Meg Turner

The odd thing for me about this piece on knowing (and not knowing) what we know is that I am now convinced that Marina somehow knew I was writing it even before *I* knew. (Such was the relationship between client and therapist.) But I could hardly have anticipated this when she first came to see me two years ago. I remember seeing this young, 23-year-old Conservatory student still tied to the themes and recollections of her adolescence, sitting quietly with her hands set apart, almost disjointedly on her lap, even though I now know her pianist's fingers to be rich with kinesthetic memories of preludes, etudes, Bach *Two- and Three-Part Inventions,* (and perhaps the Rachmaninoff concerto she has not yet allowed herself to perform). To me she had a cameo face, like someone who would find herself almost at home in a period piece, like a character in *A Room with a View* (Forster, 1989). And I remember thinking how here we both were, each struggling to translate an inner life into words and music, thereby embodying that life in even a modest way.

Meg Turner, PhD, is a developmental and clinical psychologist who is on the faculty of the Human Development and Psychology Department at the Harvard Graduate School of Education. She is a licensed practicing psychotherapist and Director of the Counseling Center at the New England Conservatory of Music. Currently she is working on combining academic and literary traditions in her writing.

I would like to acknowledge the contributions of my client and the friends and colleagues who have informed my writing.

SOMETHING OF MARINA'S FAMILY HISTORY: IMPROVISATIONS

Early on it was essential to Marina that I understand one thing: that music was what mattered to her, music was what made her feel real, music was a way of expressing herself more freely and of being known. "It gives me a more complete version of myself," she told me. "It also gives me some dignity, I think," she added. "I never feel like I'm really alive unless I play the piano."

At the same time, she told me that she had crying fits, that she was filled with anguish. She thought it had something to do with her body. She told me very carefully and convincingly that playing the piano was not about fingers, it was about being able to use your whole body. "The impulse starts in your brain and then moves throughout your entire being." But her studio instructor was telling her that she wasn't moving freely, that she was encumbered, and she herself felt separated from her body. "I want you to help me play my body into being," she told me solemnly, as if she knew from the very beginning that her sense of being alive in her music and her anguish about her body were intricately linked.

As I listened, it became clear that she felt separated not only from her own body but also from her memories, or her "rememberings," as she called them. "Instead of remembering, I create fictions. I improvise until I actually lose track of the original theme," she said, articulating a process of psychological resistance, a reluctance to know what she knew. I wondered what improvisations we might compose together, what themes we might obscure, despite our joint efforts to speak truthfully.

It seemed that much of her "improvising" had to do with her family When she was little, she thought her parents had a perfect marriage. She couldn't imagine her mother being unkind or critical. She had so carefully improvised her own rendition of the perfect family and the perfect mother that at times I think it was hard for her to discern what was and wasn't real.

As we listened to the range of Marina's improvisations, trying to discern the main themes, we discovered together that the improvisational nature of compositions made them no less real. What emerged initially for Marina was a rendition that sounded almost like a caricature of a traditional, upper middle-class family. There was the big beautiful house and garden; the perfect only child who was polite and excelled in school; the father who was the head of the household, who rarely spoke or participated but gave his wife money every month, and balanced her checkbook; and the perfect mother who had been the homecoming queen, was polite and pleasant, and wore fashionable, expensive clothes. Through this caricature of a perfect existence, perhaps Marina absorbed a family truth: appearances mattered more than feelings.

What seemed most obscured from Marina and from those around her was the reality that all the while she was growing up, Marina felt depressed and unhappy with herself. She was convinced that something was wrong with *her* since everything around her was fine.

But certain phrases didn't fit smoothly with this improvisation. Marina told me that there were no male figures in her life. "I have a father," she told me," but I'm not too close to him. My mother's more important in my development." She seemed to linger on a conversation she had with her friend Emily. Emily had confided that she did not have a father, even though Marina knew otherwise. "Maybe all you have is your soul," Marina replied, quoting a Tracy Chapman song, perhaps revealing the sense that there were ways in which her own father did not exist for her. She also disclosed that when she was little, she was always afraid of her father. She acknowledged that he was gruff ("Not like my mother, who's loving and easy to talk to"), but that he never did anything to merit this strong reaction on her part. Still, she was afraid to be alone with him because she couldn't think of anything to say, and she thought this was her fault. Marina thus began to play a new improvisation, haltingly, playing and stopping.

In a similar vein, she began to improvise new variations on the theme of her relationship with her mother. The improvisations belied her earlier rendition of the perfect, all-loving mother. She told me that, "For the longest time I couldn't make a move without my mother. When I was little, I just couldn't get enough from her." I wondered aloud about what kinds of things she had hoped to get. I wondered silently whose needs were being met, then immediately worried that I might be feeling too cynical toward Marina's mother.

Marking my own silence on this matter, I wondered about how Marina's tendency to make a modest criticism of a family member and then withdraw it, always doing and undoing, resembled my own resistance to claiming what I know. What was it that so needed to be undone? And by whom? By Marina? By me as her therapist? What were all the compositions that could not yet be known or played?

Marina told me that she used to follow her mother all around. (She said this while casting a shy, but evident glance at the picture postcard of ducklings on my bookshelf.) Apparently there was ample opportunity for "imprinting" because she stayed home from school for long stretches due to allergies. But at one point Marina's paternal grandmother observed to her daughter-in-law, "Marina doesn't seem to cough except when she's around you." In our session, Marina remembered having turned this statement around at the time so as to avoid blaming her mother. Instead, she worried that she herself might be fabricating her illnesses. As always, she was left wondering what was real. I wondered about how I could join her in the process of coming to know what she knew, whatever that might be – about her attachment, her love, her need, and even her mother's need to be followed.

Themes around needs and around whose needs were being met reemerged. (In fact, these themes were never silent in the room.) It appeared from this set of themes that Marina's mother could not tolerate a daughter who was physically and psychologically separate from herself. I had to remind myself that some people only know relationship as fusion. Marina put it succinctly, "For all intents and purposes, I was supposed to be exactly like my Mom." Over time I observed, in pieces and with many variations, that it was as if Marina's mother's need became Marina's need. First, her mother and then Marina herself, perhaps in an attempt to protect her mother and ultimately herself, had tried to make the daughter into a mirror image of the mother. It was as if to preserve her mother, Marina was willing to sacrifice herself. "I tried to save my mother's life, to keep her whole," Marina told me. Not until much later did she say, "I can't save anybody else's life. I can barely save my own." I remember feeling relieved, hearing the clarity of this new note in her voice.

But the familiar themes often drowned out the new notes. It seemed that Marina's mother had countless ways (all born of her own need, of course, but no less compelling for Marina) of seducing Marina into giving birth to a replica of her mother. Marina told me that her mother would say things like, "The way you treat me is how your children will treat you," and "When you suffer, I suffer too. And I'm getting older. It hurts me more than it hurts you."

As we listened to these maxims together, we both came to know that however much Marina loved her mother, it would never be enough ("She loved so much, she could not love enough," was how Marina put it, describing her fantasy of Clara Schumann). Marina could not become her mother and survive as herself.

THE MAIN THEME: RESIDING IN "THE BETWEEN"

With this new clarity, I began to wonder if for the timeless years before I knew her, Marina resided asymptotically close to two poles of human existence, poles so extreme that each was an almost unimaginable theoretical abstraction of attachment and loss: absolute merger and absolute isolation.

The only way that her mother could allow the two of them to be in a relationship together was via merger, so extreme a form of connection that it cannot be termed a relationship. The only allowable alternative for Marina seemed to be total isolation. In this regard, the emotional meaning underlying Marina's appropriation of her mother's spoken and unspoken messages seemed unambiguous: "To the extent that you are a body, a separate being, you are other than me and therefore bad." And so Marina lived in fear of being alienated from her mother, "The division into despair," as she called it, recalling Dostoevsky's (1968) *Notes from the Underground.* This division meant that she would be exiled, that she would have her own body, but that having a body would itself be repugnant. In essence, *she* would be repugnant.

Working together, we constructed and deconstructed the chords of some of Marina's deepest emotional truths. Thinking of her allusion to "the division into despair," I had my own associations and was reminded that I had my own chords to deconstruct. I thought of the traditional psychoanalytic, structural notion that the development of the self depends on a separation or differentiation from the other as well as on a differentiation of one internal structure from the other. For example, according to Loewald (1978), Freud described the superego as a "differentiating grade in the ego" (p. 24). Thinking more about this differentiating grade in the ego, I recalled Grosz's (1990) reference to "Lacan's conception of the ego as *inherently* alienated" (p. 48). I puzzled over the metaphor of alienation and looked to Grosz and Loewald for clarification. Grosz (1990) told me that "The ego is split, internally divided between self and other" (p. 47). Loewald (1978) told me that "I believe that Lacan's idea of the ego as a structure of alienation is related to the splitting in which duality becomes established" (p. 41). It seems that for Loewald and for the Lacanian psychoanalyst Schneiderman (cited in Ragland-Sullivan, 1986), *splitting* can refer to the split between conscious and unconscious process or meaning. Further, Loewald, for example, does not stop here but acknowledges that splitting and duality "make possible a *conscire*, a knowing together" (p. 41). Even so, I was left with the idea of internal splits or splits between the self and others.

I felt as if I were selectively attending to metaphors that I found unsettling. Dostoevsky spoke of *division,* Loewald spoke of *splitting,* Lacanians spoke of *alienation* and *splitting*. I knew that there were certainly ways in which these same authors also spoke of relationship, but when I thought of Marina's allusion to despair, I found myself wanting to emphasize relationship even more. I wanted to italicize the idea that this division or this alienation or this splitting then serves as a basis for relatedness not only to oneself but also to others. "The self is a relation which relates itself to its own self" Kierkegaard (1954, p. 146) tells me. But beyond this solipsism, what about relationships? As Cole (1971) has indicated, both Kierkegaard and Freud implied that for the potential self to grow and become a self, it must first relate itself to something outside of itself. Or, as my work with Marina helped me voice the theme: "Is there a way to use difference as a basis for authentic relationships?"

This question hung in the air as the therapy continued. Marina felt caught on the horns of a dilemma. If she identified with her mother to the point of functional merger, then she would be refusing to know what she knew: the reality of her own existence, the fact that she was "a creature with a name" (Becker, 1973, p. 3), the fact that she had her own body and bodily desires. This choice would be tantamount to an affirmation of nonexistence. At the same time, if she refused to merge with her mother, then, since even minute differences led to total isolation in her mother's eyes (and Marina was exquisitely attuned to the reflection in her mother's eyes as well as mine), it would be as if she chose a kind of existence in which she was repugnant, alien, and alone. And what kind of existence would that be? It felt like another form of nonexistence to Marina. The two poles, the two horns of Marina's dilemma, were ironically close together.

At times it was as if Marina felt "condemned to choice" (Valle & King, 1978, p. 8) as she alternated between poles, going from one to the other, doing and undoing. But more often she resided in "the between" (Prescott & Valle, 1978, p. 159), caught in the dialectical tension between the two, fighting for more air, while feeling at once bound to her mother and alien, even repugnant. And her allergies continued. "It's hard to play the piano if you can't breathe," she would tell me, "and playing the piano is as much about breathing as it is about fingers." At such times I would silently think of Milan Kundera's (1984) description of Stalin's son:

> Who ran to electrocute himself on the barbed wire when he could no longer stand to watch the poles of human existence come so close to each other as to touch. (p. 268)

VARIATIONS ON THE THEME IN ADOLESCENCE: RETROSPECTIVES

I shudder now as I think of how the poles of existence made themselves felt to Marina in the years before I knew her. To the extent that she became her mother and part of the family and culture that had borne her mother, Marina could not have a body or bodily desires, since a body would designate her as separate from her mother. "I was brought up to have no sexuality," Marina told me. At the same time, to the extent that she did allow herself her bodily existence along with its desires, both she and her desires were bad. "My mother taught me that sex was really bad. The message was, 'Be desired but don't have desires yourself.' "

Thinking back, she was convinced that she had always felt that something was wrong with her physically. "Something about my genitals was wrong," she told me, although it was difficult for her to clarify just what. Even her earliest memory, from about the age of three, embodied this concern:

> I remember my mother becoming sort of upset because I had some sort of a diaper rash or something. She was totally alarmed and called my father, "Jeffrey, Jeffrey, come here and look at this."

Marina described "a whole horror I had of my body since I was little," but it seems that the complexities of her relationship to her body intensified in high school, a time when, in her terms, she felt "out of control." During this period she mustered the courage to ask her mother about her body. She needed to know if her body was all right or not, if she was normal. But Marina said that her mother dismissed her concerns without pause, "Oh, of course it's fine." Marina was not consoled.

In large part Marina felt dissociated from her body, ignoring its existence; and the times when she did acknowledge that she had a body, she felt repulsion or disgust toward herself. As I heard her descriptions, I became further convinced that there is an important distinction between simply *having* a body and *being* a body: there's a more intimate relationship implicit in being than in having. I thought back to graduate school and how I had surprised myself with the staunchness of my insistence that I preserve this intimacy by translating the phenomenological world of the *Umwelt* (May, cited in Keen, 1978) in terms of "being a body in space" (Keen, 1978, p. 242). Now, thinking of the young woman before me, I understood my conviction more explicitly, and I wondered how often Marina had felt herself to be a body in space.

Her mother's edicts about sexuality only heightened Marina's tendencies to dissociate from or be repelled by her body and all bodily desires:

> If you had sex, you were a fallen woman. If you were married, you weren't supposed to like it. My mother disapproved of anyone who had sex. It was a moralizing, explicit thing from my mother.

If sex was bad, then getting pregnant was worse. Marina was certain that she would be disowned if indeed she became pregnant. As she described it,

> You could fall from grace at any moment. Even though I'd been in a state of grace up to that point [high school], I was afraid I just couldn't keep on. If I suddenly made the wrong move and didn't know it, I could be banished. If I got pregnant, I could be cast off on the street. The thought was too terrible for my parents to even mention. Sex at all was bad, but pregnancy was unthinkable.

It wasn't surprising that from the age of 12 Marina had nightmares about getting pregnant. As she described it, repeatedly in these dreams, "I hide it from my mother. I don't know how I've gotten pregnant. My parents are forcing me to have an abortion."

In our work together, Marina speculated about the source of this taboo against being sexual, a taboo linked with the risk of pregnancy and the possibility of giving birth. For her mother, giving birth seemingly meant giving birth to a mirror image of herself. As Marina described it, "My mother didn't want to accept that I was an individual. I was supposed to be a reflection of her, and that was her project." However, Marina knew that if she herself were to become pregnant, then the situation would have a different meaning and would only serve to separate her further from her mother. As she put it, "If I really gave birth, I would be giving birth to difference, and so giving birth would not be allowed." No doubt she was right because for her mother, alternatives to merger, such as difference, simply were not tolerated and in fact seemed perilous.

This fear of pregnancy translated to a more general fear of any embodied desire, whether it had to do with music (her first love after her mother) or with her sexuality. For some time Marina had been attracted to pictures of women, but it seems that in high school both the need and the reluctance to know what she knew in this regard became especially acute. As she told me in retrospect:

Marina: Especially when I was younger, I had sexual feelings and impulses, but I just never let myself acknowledge them.

Me: What happened to all those feelings?

Marina: I felt the most out of control in high school. I was trying to deny my needs, my response to women.

Me: Were you alone with that?

Marina: I couldn't tell anyone. In high school I jumped from masturbating and not realizing the connection to women, to looking at a woman. I was in quite a struggle there. I thought it was awful. I went for a long time without making it conscious. Then I couldn't deny what was happening any more. I made the conscious resolution that no one in the world had to know but me. No one would ever know. I could hide it so well. If I couldn't overcome it, I could hide it very well. I wasn't allowing it to *be*. But then I was over at a friend's house. I tried not to see women naked. I avoided it–it would make it too horrible. It was hard enough if people were clothed. We were watching this film that had nude women. I couldn't bolt. I couldn't just leave. I had to stay there and experience the horror of it. I cried the first time when I didn't want anyone to know. I could never tell my mother. I wanted my mother to tell me it was okay, this too shall pass.

I was filled with the sense of her agony and courage, as I followed her initial reluctance to know what she knew into her even greater reluctance to tell what she knew. I wondered how I could be there with her now in ways that would be different for her. How could we make a safe place for her in the room, a room set apart from a homophobic culture, a room where whatever Marina knew could be safely told?

To some extent music had helped Marina express all that she knew. As she put it, "Through music I can release myself from being really blocked." In essence, music preserved some of her desire. But at the same time, she knew that to be a pianist she must also be a body. Thus, implicit in every theme she played was the same dialectic: How to be at once tied to her mother but with a body and a being of her own? Again, given the context of her history, being a separate body meant being repugnant in some sense. With her music, this meant that she continually devalued her playing. She worried constantly about betraying the composer by failing to do justice to the work. At the same time, if, in her frustration, she gave up playing all together, relinquishing her music and all that it meant to her, then it would be as if she were condemning herself to a kind of nonexistence. At the very least, giving up music would symbolize the death of her own desire. It seemed that there was no way out of this dialectic save through the illusory power of her mind. For Marina, thought became an antidote to desire. She convinced herself that if she just thought hard enough, things would be okay. She allowed herself and others to be seduced by good grades, but inwardly she felt torn at best, numb at worst.

TRANSFORMATIONS OF THE THEME IN YOUNG ADULTHOOD

By the time Marina first presented herself in my office, her relationship to her music and to people outside of her family had already helped her to find ways of expressing much of what had been unspoken as an adolescent. However, while the internalized voices associated with her dialectical theme, or with the horns of her dilemma, were now more distinct, they still needed to be heard relative to one another and orchestrated as a whole.

My relationship with Marina involved a continual orchestration of the voices of intimacy and separateness, making it possible for Marina to know what she knew. I felt more confident about this orchestration when Marina brought in a dream fragment: "I was taking off my clothes in a haphazard way. I asked you, 'Is my body all right?' I was showing you my body."

When I inquired about her feelings in the dream, she told me that she had felt affirmed by me. I was grateful that she had not felt dismissed as she had when she asked her mother the same question. Marina was bringing more of herself into the room and was orchestrating more of what she knew. Increasingly I was aware that what she knew was not restricted to her own history but touched on mine as well. My first awareness of this likelihood came when she related the following dream: "We were trying to talk to each other from different rooms. We couldn't really see each other, but we were trying to communicate. Then I could see both of us."

The dream was rich with possible meanings, but what I focused on internally was the last sentence, the idea that she could see both of us, that she knew something about both of us. What and how much could she see I wondered? What was she seeing or hearing that I was missing? What was my own reluctance to know keeping me from knowing about myself and about Marina?

A few months later, Marina related another dream:

> I had a dream about therapy. It was about you and not you. I had an appointment with a therapist. She was supposed to be you. She was dressed like you, but she was my age, my contemporary. She wouldn't sit down – we had to go somewhere else. She took me around Boston. I kept waiting to start. Why were we going around? I was anxious, anticipating. I thought she was going to tell me something about herself. It was an intense thing. I was intent on following her around, on talking to her finally. Maybe we went back to the original room. I thought she might tell me why we were going around or that she might reveal something about herself. I felt trusted.

This dream seems to me to be a request, a wish that I bring myself more fully and authentically into my relationship with Marina. Particularly in light of this wish, it amazes me that in our exploration of this dream I neglected to ask what the therapist in her dream might have revealed. How was it that I could have avoided this question? Was there something I knew she knew about me which I was afraid to acknowledge about myself? In the words of her dream, "Why were we going around" instead of getting to the heart of what we both knew?

Ironically, I had seen myself as joining in her efforts to know what she knew, as she was ready to know it. But now I wonder if I was simultaneously neglecting my own reluctance to know what I knew: both something about myself and something essential about her, namely, the extent to which she could discern things about me, the extent to which she needed to know who I was, what I knew.

But why was I afraid to hear what she could discern about me, the kernel of truth in her projections or in her accurate perceptions? Did I fear becoming too real, not only to her but to myself? Could it be that I was avoiding the ways in which aspects of her struggle mirrored my own? While Marina was working to orchestrate her internalized voices, I too was working to construct a different, more fully textured and embodied voice, and a name that is more fully my own. Simply put, I wanted to be able to speak and write in the first person, and to sign the work with a name that felt more like my own.

"Naming names," I remembered was the title of a chapter by novelist John Hawkes (1963-1964, p. 1). Naming myself seemed like such an immediate and personal form of appropriation. In one breath it balances the separateness implicit in having a name of my own and the relatedness implicit in being accessible through my name and therefore potentially knowable. I can use a name to hide behind or to be known. But as I sat with Marina in the nestled room that is my office, I found myself wanting to be known more, that is, wanting to bring myself more authentically into our relationship. I wanted to know more of what I knew and to hear more of what Marina knew.

I hear the ways in which Marina is implicitly a truthteller. I know she knows things her mother couldn't allow herself to know explicitly (for example, that Marina is a sexual being). I know too that Marina knows things she's afraid I can't hear. And some of her dreams tell me that she knew I might be writing about us even before *I* knew.

As I became more sensitive in my listening for what Marina and I had left unspoken, the things I had been reluctant to know, Marina seemed to say more and to reframe the phrasing of her own struggle. This mature and accomplished pianist went back to practicing the simplest of Bach's *Two-Part Inventions*. The problem, as she described it, was that she hadn't distinguished each of the two voices adequately in the context of the other. Her strategy seemed straightforward: she was to separate the hands, playing one voice on the piano while singing the other voice. In this way, each voice could be distinguished in relation to the other – one played, the other sung. Given that she was right-handed, she was surprised to find that her left hand seemed to have a broader range of expression in this endeavor, that it sounded more solid and even, and tapered more gracefully at the ends of phrases.

We came to hear this distinction between her right and left hands as a metaphor for the ways in which she felt separated from herself and her body. "My right hand has a certain technical precision," she told me, "but it sounds too exact, almost measured. It's all fingers. My left hand sounds softer, freer, darker, warmer. It feels more connected to the rest of my body. But now that my hands are more distinguishable, I have to find a way to coordinate them, while preserving something of each. They're two hands, but they're also of one body." I recalled how at the start of therapy, she had wanted me to help her play her body into being. Thinking of Dallery (1989) and the French feminist Cixous (1981), I thought too of how much I wanted to write my body into being, by finding an embodied voice.

During this period there were times when Marina practiced so relentlessly that there was a tightening in her muscles. It felt as if too much was asked in trying to coordinate the differing textures of both hands: "Too much courage," she told me. I wondered how much courage would be asked of each of us separately and together.

But as Marina struggled to coordinate her left hand with the right, she became increasingly connected to her body. Together we continued to explore themes around her sexuality, and she began to clarify the development of her own desire. This exploration was partly inspired by a reading assignment in one of her humanities courses: some feminist criticism on Louisa May Alcott's (1947) book, *Little Women*. Marina thought of the close relationship the daughters (Meg, Jo, Beth, and Amy) had with their mother, Marmee, and of her own close relationship with her mother. She thought back to when she was little: "I used to like having my mother there alone, with no father. I was secretly glad when he was away on business." But then her tone darkened: "It's hard when your mother is the first person you love, and then you must also separate from her," she told me. Marina sounded impassioned: "In some ways it seems absurd to prescribe heterosexuality after a homoerotic relationship with the mother. This was Jo's problem. She was forced into heterosexuality and was never satisfied."

Marina then began analyzing Meg. I smile at these words as I read what I have just written. In fourth grade, when someone asked if "Meg" was short for "Marjorie," I surprised myself by asserting definitively, "No, it's another name for 'Margaret.'" Was it then that I first silently took the name *Meg*, defining myself as distinct from my family, who called me "Margaret," by beginning to name myself? I remember whispering "Meg."

But in the midst of my associations, Marina was still talking about Meg and the kiss on Meg's wedding day. I was puzzled by her reference and feared I had missed something, so that night, I consulted my well-worn copy of *Little Women.* I found the description of Meg's wedding ceremony, and the reference became clear:

> It wasn't all the thing, I'm afraid, but the minute she was fairly married, Meg cried, "The first kiss for Marmee!" and, turning, gave it with her heart on her lips. (Alcott, 1947, p. 279)

I thought of merger, of being married to one's mother as it were, and of its dialectical opposite, isolation. I realized that Marina was neither merged with her mother nor isolated, and I marveled at the ways in which she was placing herself as separate but always in relation to others. She was no longer simply taking what was given but was constructing and claiming what she needed to be authentic.

And at some point, I realized that Marina was playing the Bach *Two-Part Invention* with both hands, each voiced separately, with a different texture, but always in relation to the other and to the whole of the piece. It was as if, through the music, she was slowly and quickly playing her body into being, thereby giving birth to herself.

For my part, I decided that it was time to try my hand at writing in the first person.

LEAVING AND UNLEAVING

As Marina's hands came to play more of what she knew, she became increasingly preoccupied with mortality and with the finiteness of the body. Themes of loss permeated the hour. "I don't know if I can bear to watch another season change," she told me. "Everything seems too green." I thought of T. S. Eliot's (1971) description of April:

> April is the cruellest month, breeding
> Lilacs out of the dead land, mixing
> Memory and desire, stirring
> Dull roots with spring rain. (p. 37)

But Marina had her own associations. She thought of Gerard Manley Hopkins' (1985) poem, "Spring and Fall: To a Young Child." She quoted the first two lines:

> Margaret, are you grieving
> Over Goldengrove unleaving? (p. 50)

I paused, surprised because these were among my favorite lines. "Margaret;" I said, thinking of the transference. "Oh, I hadn't noticed that it began with 'Margaret,' " she said. "I don't attach that name to you." She has always called me "Dr. Turner." Whatever she called me, I heard these lines as if Marina were speaking directly to me, as if she were naming me.

As she associated to the poem, she told me that given the fact of mortality, she wanted to live life as consciously as possible, "Like Debussy, making music, so that at least at moments it's like the world opening up." I thought of Freud inviting us to make what is unconscious conscious (cited in Loewald, 1978). I heard Marina's words to mean that she wanted to know and tell what she knows and that there would be music in the telling.

As I write this piece, I think of my own process of coming to know what I know, of Hawkes' (1963-1964, p. 1) notion of "naming names." I know that there are ways in which I still name myself after the Meg in *Little Women* and the Margaret born of my reading of "Spring and Fall." I think of Marina's allusions to "Meg," who is so bound to her mother, and to "Margaret," who is in a sense so separate because of her attunement to loss. I am especially drawn to Margaret. Like Margaret and Marina, I hate to see the seasons change. I mourn the fact that people must leave and trees must unleave. I mourn the fact of mortality itself. As Hopkins (1985) knew,

> It is the blight man was born for,
> It is Margaret you mourn for. (p. 50)

But while reflecting on Marina's allusions to "Meg" and "Margaret," I realize that I am also different from both of them. And at long last, I allow myself to know what I have known implicitly all along, namely, my name. It is the name I whispered to myself in fourth grade, a name of my choosing – tied to my family and to literature, but still my own. I realize too that my relationship with Marina has helped me to know more of what I know, that she has helped to name me.

CODA

I still find it odd to think that Marina somehow knew I was writing this piece even before *I* knew. The first time I got a conscious sense that this might be so was actually a few months before I had even been approached about writing something about women and therapy. Marina brought me a dream she'd had while staying with friends. In the dream I dedicated two books to her, one on music, the other on psychology. I remember feeling both surprised and embarrassed gratified when she told me. Had she perceived my involvement in music, my own (unrealized) dream of becoming a concert pianist, much as she was struggling to become one now? Was she unconsciously attuned to my longing to write, a longing so secret that only rarely did I let myself know it? At the time I don't think I would have consciously given voice to the wish to write such a piece: I was feeling torn between the need to remain private and silent on the one hand, and the longing for relationship via expression on the other. My struggle mirrored Marina's struggle to define herself authentically. Her struggle involved considerable dissonance (so much so that she often questioned the possibility and even the concept of resolution) since, to some extent, authenticity meant having to define herself as different from a family and culture which, in combination with her history, were keeping her from having more authentic relationships with herself, with people she cared about, and with her own body.

Once I had already started writing this piece and was going back over my notes, I discovered that for at least a year Marina had this implicit knowledge about my desire to write, a desire that I was only now allowing myself to know. Although happily versed in Searles' (1979) article on "The Patient as Therapist to His Analyst," I still found myself marveling at how it was that she could know more about me than I could let myself know about myself. Was it the interplay (and ultimately the harmony) between her obvious attunement to – yet distinctiveness from – me that allowed her to know what she knew? I puzzled. Still, the evidence seemed clear. A year earlier she had brought me the following dream:

> We were in closer physical proximity. You showed me a book you'd written. You were the author of a book called, *In the Ear of the Other,* based on a text by Derrida [1982/1985] which my first piano teacher had given me. You confided that the critics didn't understand it.

But such open expression, the willingness to know what we know, seemed like such a revealing and therefore potentially hazardous enterprise to each of us. As Marina once disclosed, "My private things are like little demons." At the same time, I suggested to her that she took pleasure in these little demons, much the way she relished the slight mistranslation of the Prokofiev piece she was practicing, *Suggestion Diabolique* ("Devilish Inspiration").

Certainly each of us, albeit in the context of our private fears, consciously and unconsciously flirted with and was inspired by what seemed like the unspeakable or even the unknowable in our lives. And while the contexts of our lives differed, for each of us the question was essentially the same: How were we to allow ourselves to know what we know and to do so publicly, whether in music or in words?

REFERENCES

Alcott, L. M. (1947). *Little women.* New York: Grosset & Dunlap.

Becker, E. (1973). *The denial of death.* New York: The Free Press.

Cixous, H. (1981). The laugh of the Medusa. In E. Marks & I. de Courtivron (Eds.), *New French feminisms: An anthology* (pp. 245-264). New York: Schocken Books. (Original work [Le rire de la meduse] published in 1975)

Cole, J. P. (1971). *The problematic self in Kierkegaard and Freud.* New Haven: Yale University Press.

Dallery, A. (1989). The politics of writing (the) body: *Ecriture feminine.* In A. Jaggar & S. Bordo (Eds.), *Gender/body/knowledge: Feminist reconstructions of being and knowing* (pp. 52-67). New Brunswick, NJ: Rutgers University Press.

Derrida, J. (1985). Otobiographies: The teaching of Nietssche and the politics of the proper name (A. Ronell, Trans.). In C. McDonald (Ed.) and P. Kamuf (Trans.), *The ear of the other: Otobiography, transference, translation: Texts and discussions with Jacques Derrida.* New York: Schocken Books. (Original work [L'oreille de l'autre] published in 1982)

Dostoevsky, F. (1968). Notes from the underground. In *Great short works of Dostoevsky* (pp. 263-377). New York: Harper & Row. (Original work published in 1864)

Eliot, T. S. (1971). "The burial of the dead" from The waste land. In *The complete poems and plays 1909-1950* (pp. 37-39). San Diego: Harcourt Brace Jovanovich. (Original work published in 1922)

Forster, E. M. (1989). *A room with a view.* New York: Vintage International. (Original work published in 1923)

Grosz, E. (1990). *Jacques Lacan: A feminist introduction.* New York: Routledge.

Hawkes, J. (1963-1964). *Second skin.* New York: New Directions.

Hopkins, G. M. (1985). "Spring and Fall: To a Young Child." In W. H. Gardner (Ed.), *Poems and prose of Gerard Manly Hopkins* (p. 50). New York: Viking Penguin Inc. (Original work published in 1918)

Keen, E. (1978). Psychopathology. In R. S. Valle & M. King (Eds.), *Existentialpl-lenomenological alternatives for psychology* (pp. 234-264). New York: Oxford University Press.

Kierkegaard, S. (1954). *The sickness unto death.* (W. Lowrie, Trans.). Princeton, NJ: Princeton University Press. (Original Work published in 1849)

Kundera, M. (1984). *The unbearable lightness of being.* New York: Harper & Row.

Loewald, H. (1978). *Psychoanalysis and the history of the individual.* New Haven: Yale University Press.

Prescott, M. P., & Valle, R. S. (1978). An existential-phenomenological look at cognitive-developmental theory and research. In R. S. Valle & M. King (Eds.), *Existential-phenomenological alternatives for psychology* (pp. 153-165). New York: Oxford University Press.

Ragland-Sullivan, E. (1986). *Jacques Lacan and the philosophy of psychoanalysis.* Urbana and Chicago, IL: University of Illinois Press.

Searles, H. F. (1979). The patient as therapist to his analyst. In H. Searles (Ed.), *Countertransference and related subjects* (pp. 380-459). New York: International Universities Press.

Valle, R. S., & King, M. (1978). An introduction to existential-phenomenological thought in psychology. In R. S. Valle & M. King (Eds.), *Existential-phenomenological alternatives for psychology* (pp. 6-17). New York: Oxford University Press.

The Body at Play

Elizabeth Debold

In my mind's eye, at the top left comer of this page is a photograph taken of my brother and me–although, it would be more accurate to forswear grammar and say "me and my brother" because it's me at 11 (so my brother's 10). I remember the photograph vividly even though the colors of the film are now ghostly pale. That photograph belongs in this story. Through the memory of the photograph I began to remember that time.

I have a story to tell. Woven through time, twisted on itself and doubled like a strand of DNA, this story is a story of psychic life inscribed in my body. I lived this story as it lived me for more than twenty years before I knew it–in part by remembering it and in part by seeing it happen again in the lives of other girls and women. The research of Carol Gilligan, Lyn Mikel Brown and my other colleagues at the Harvard Project on the Psychology of Women and the Development of Girls intertwined with the story of my memory, leading me to return to my own life to search for the feelings of myself as a girl before I reconstructed myself as a woman. In telling this story, I wish to flesh out my thinking and explore how women literally embody ideas of womanhood.

This work is set against the background of recent writings that explore, to use the title of Susan Suleiman's (1986) volume, "the female body in Western culture." Through innumerable words and images, both sacred and profane, Western culture presents woman's

---

Elizabeth Debold is a member of the Harvard Project on the Psychology of Women and the Development of Girls. She is currently studying embodied knowledge and the mind/body split in adolescent girls.

body as possessing the power to deliver and devour life, "a source of pleasure and nurturance, but also of destruction and evil. Mary and Pandora, in sum" (p. 1). The lips that speak, the eyes that see, the hand that writes or draws these representations of the female body belong to men, literally or figuratively, the creators of Western culture. Suleiman's project is to consider "the cultural significance of the female body [which] is not only (not even first and foremost), that of a flesh-and-blood entity, but that of a *symbolic construct*" (p. 2, emphasis in original).

I would like to stand Suleiman's project on its head and ask, given the symbolic construct of the female body as a source of pleasure and danger, what does this mean to the "flesh-and-blood entity"? If women's sexuality is defined by the pleasure and fear aroused by women's bodies which, in turn, may make sexuality dangerous to women themselves, what happens, then, to the play of feelings in girls' bodies as they move into adolescence? If women's sexuality–a powerful part of bodily experience–is constructed as problematic or illicit, then might not this result in women experiencing discomfort or disease in their bodies?

Recently, I asked my mother for that photograph. "You're wearing a plaid shirt and blue shorts," she said immediately. She remembered as well. She had made my outfit. "Why do you want that one?" she asked. A good question since in the photograph I'm standing in the front yard at a batting tee, holding the baseball bat rigidly, my arms bent at right angles like Gumby. I'm wearing a grimace of a smile for my father who thinks he's taking a photograph of his daughter who, with her perfect batting stance, will be the first girl in Little League (in 1966!). No surprise that my brother looks caught somewhere between listlessness and sheer discomfort. (My brother was a gifted ballplayer.)

I told my mother that the photograph represented a real conflict for me. A sound indicating comprehension and utter indignation clicked in her throat. "I ***hated*** *when your father did that to you," she said, "You didn't like playing baseball."*

In 1895, Freud also "enter[s] into a girl's feelings" (1895/1955, p. 144) to tell the story of another Elizabeth, in the case of Fraulein Elisabeth von R. (at least as presented in the Standard English Edition, translated by James Strachey in collaboration with Anna Freud). He tells us of Elisabeth's playful relationship with her father and characterizes the play in bodily terms: her father "jokingly called her 'cheeky' and 'cock-sure'" (p. 140). Elisabeth's desire for love is played out in pains in her legs so severe that "'standing alone' [was] painful to her" (p. 152). Elisabeth finds herself as a young woman in nursing her father until his death, caring for her mother throughout her illnesses, and standing helplessly at the deathbed of her sister. Yet, Elisabeth also begins to find in her own body a "restless, yearning mood" which shows that, in a sense, she is of two hearts (p. 151). Her bodily pain begins as her love for her mother and sister is joined by a love that she cannot acknowledge–her love for her brother-in-law, that is, her sister's husband.

Freud (again in the English translation) characterizes Elisabeth's feelings of yearning, of warmth, of burning in unabashedly, and at the same time, innocently sexual terms. And yet, he seems to look away from Elisabeth's body, as if averting his eyes from the place, the site, where this burning and yearning is happening. Freud helps Elisabeth to understand that her idea that her feelings were "such wickedness"–leading to an impasse in her body's movement–can also be understood as a desire for love, the foundation of human goodness (p. 157).

> *My friend M. called me one day last summer to tell me of a dream. It takes place on the edge of an expanse of water. She recognized as parts of herself the two children looking into the water. There was an older, naked adolescent self and a 10-year-old self. The 10-year-old nearly drowns while rescuing the older self's clothing from sinking below the surface of the water.*
>
> *We were both struck by the 10-year-old's ability to act, particularly when contrasted with the naked vulnerability of the older adolescent. We began talking about the activity of being 10 and 11: fearlessly roller-skating down hills, diving into wa-*

> *ter, running flat out in foot races. M. remembered beating her brother in a foot race. Once I beat Joey, who was supposed to be really fast. The older boys on the block demanded that we run it again: I wouldn't. M.'s father taught her to catch a football. Mine did too. I remembered catching a baseball with him, too. The ball made a heavy sound when it slammed into the pocket of my mitt. My hand would sting. I liked it.*

In fifth grade, age 10, Victoria's vision is acute. Victoria, part of a longitudinal study of girls attending a private girls' school in the Midwest directed by Lyn Mikel Brown and Carol Gilligan, wonders at what is happening in her mother's life. She notices that "everything always points to the man, like the man is most important and the woman is not even alive." She worries for her mother because, if her parents

> got a divorce, and she had to go to work no one would know who she was, they would just, even if they knew her, just from like seeing the couple, you know, my mom and dad together, they would always think of her as Mrs. Whatever.

Overhearing ominous discussions between her parents, Victoria begins to think about what it means for her mother to be a woman in a culture where "the men always think they're better."

Yet, despite the clarity of her vision, Victoria is haunted by the specter of what Lyn Mikel Brown (1989) calls "the perfect girl." Now, in sixth grade, she says that she used to feel panicky if she did something bad because "if I got yelled at then I knew I wasn't perfect." Lyn Brown has noticed that, beginning in the fifth grade, these girls censor themselves to appear more like "the nice and perfect girl who has no bad thoughts" and who is the girl that adult women seem to prefer (p. 113). This self-censoring of thought and action begins to double girls' vision: one way of looking shows them the image of the perfect girl in her perfect life while the other way of looking, which often becomes cloudy at puberty, shows them what they know from experience – that "the woman is not even alive."

> *The photograph came to my mind. What is hidden in the picture is my mother, standing behind the screen door frantically stage-whispering to my father, "You're ruining that girl's life. You're going to ruin her life." I had no idea what that meant. But, gradually, a haze of self-consciousness, a vague fear, cast a shadow over my body. I felt awkward playing catch. I looked like Gumby at the bat. I began to run "like a girl." I stayed in the house and read books. I was perfectly well-behaved.*

Across the seas of time and culture, Jamaica Kincaid (1985b) captures, in a short piece entitled "Girl," the instructions and warnings given to a girl as her body changes her into a young woman. The unmistakable voice of a mother patters like sharp rain on a roof, slightly irritating yet comforting to those warm inside:

> this is how you sweep a corner; this is how you sweep a whole house; this is how you sweep a yard; this is how you smile to someone you don't like too much; this is how you smile to someone you don't like at all; this is how you smile to someone you like completely; . . . this is how to behave in the presence of men who don't know you very well, and this way they won't recognize immediately the slut I have warned you against becoming; be sure to wash every day, even if it is with your own spit; don't squat down to play marbles–you are not a boy, you know. . . .(pp. 4-5)

Across the divide of puberty, the simple childhood play of the daughter–singing, walking, eating fruit on the street, playing marbles–is renamed by this mother as carelessness or, perhaps even worse, as "boy" behavior. The unconscious, loose limbed movements of the girl are an invitation to play; those movements in a young woman are another kind of invitation. Sexuality opens the daughter to the possibility of love as well as the danger of being labelled a "slut." The mother's words of warning about unspoken yet clear danger now circumscribe the play of this girl's body.

> *M. and I wanted to go bike riding but rain the next morning washed out our plans. I suggested that we go to the store and get stuff to play with when the sun came out. I wanted to play catch.*

Jerome Kagan (1972) listens to the responses of two fifteen-year-old girls describing how their ideas of "growing up" alter their play after they begin menstruating. "It was like growing up over night," says the first girl about crossing the divide into womanhood, "I felt like I was not a little kid anymore. I couldn't ride my bicycle anymore; really I'm not kidding you." The interviewer asks her if she was happy: "No, but I just thought I was above riding a bicycle or playing with dolls." The second girl makes a similar observation for herself: "I started thinking that I couldn't ride my bike and couldn't do things that made me look like a baby" (p. 97). These girls equate menstruation with becoming a woman and play with childhood: The two are mutually exclusive.

> *Before we met at the sporting goods store, I called my parents'house to get advice on buying a baseball mitt. My mother seemed puzzled and overly amused as she handed the phone to my father. He was delighted as though it was almost ordinary that his 33-year-old daughter would be buying a baseball mitt. He gave me several pointers: you catch with your longest finger on the outside of the mitt; make sure that you can easily open and close the mitt; get a mitt with a big enough pocket to be able to hold a softball. He told me not to begin by trying to throw too far. Take it easy. I hung up feeling exuberant.*

Standing at the crossroads between childhood and adulthood, in a land where the signposts all bear men's names, are a mother and her daughter. Two novels set at that crossroads, in this land, tell the story of two different girls as they take the map given to them by their mothers to begin their journey. In both Marguerite Duras's (1986) *The Lover* and Jamaica Kincaid's (1985a) *Annie John*, the transformations of the daughter's body transforms the relationship between mother and daughter. Mother becomes other as the daughter journeys into a world of sexual desire. As the unnamed girl in Duras's story realizes the power that her still child-like body gives her with men, she crosses into territory unknown to her mother, and, in so doing loses all connection with her. As Duras writes:

> I looked at my mother, I could hardly recognize her. And then, in a kind of sudden vanishing, a sudden fall, I all at once couldn't recognize her at all. There, suddenly, close to me, was someone sitting in my mother's place who wasn't my mother, who looked like her but who had never been her. . . . she was sitting just where my mother had been sitting when the substitution took place, . . . I knew no one else was there in her place, but that that identity irreplaceable by any other had disappeared and I was powerless to make it come back . . . . I did cry out. (pp. 85-86)

As the girl plays with her sexuality, her mother is lost. The daughter in the story begins to dream of death.

As Annie John's body changes, her mother changes: It was as if her mother, the love of her life, "had suddenly turned into a crocodile" (p. 84). After her mother sees her talking to boys and tells her that she was ashamed to see her daughter "behave in the manner of a slut," Annie John "save[d] myself, I turned to her and said, 'Well, like father like son, like mother like daughter'" (p. 102). This is insult, not kinship. Annie John becomes sick, depressed, and unable to move for months. After she recovers, she leaves her mother:

> Why, I wonder, didn't I see the hypocrite in my mother when, over the years, she said that she loved me and could hardly live without me, while at the same time proposing and arranging separation after separation, including this one, which, unbeknownst to her, I have arranged to be permanent? So now I, too, have hypocrisy, and breasts (small ones), and hair growing in the appropriate places, and sharp eyes, and I have made a vow never to be fooled again. (p. 133)

Annie John's small breasts cost her the paradise of childhood play with her mother.

> *Wave upon wave of anxiety, like an electric current, rushed from my feet to the top of my head as I approached the sporting goods store. My breathing became shallow, panicky. I felt dizzy and lightheaded. Keeping my awareness in the jagged flutter of my breath as it moved in and out of me, I began to be able to observe these periodic assaults as they flooded my body. My body was in acute alarm.*

In Amy Tan's (1989) *The Joy Luck Club*, a Chinese mother painfully notes her daughter's inability to speak up for herself: "If she doesn't speak, she is making a choice. If she doesn't try, she can lose her chance forever" (p. 133). The mother continues,

> I know this, because I was raised the Chinese way: I was taught to desire nothing, to swallow other people's misery, to eat my own bitterness. And even though I taught my daughter the opposite, she came out the same way! Maybe it is because she was born to me and she was born a girl. And I was born to my mother and I was born a girl. All of us are like stairs, one step after another, going up and down, but all going the same way. (p. 241)

Somehow, despite being told to be different, the daughter becomes the woman of "the Chinese way" that her mother embodies: Without desire or voice.

> *With my consciousness split between breathing to keep me from panicking and an effort to appear like any other shopper, I found M in a baseball cap and a Chicago jacket tossing a ball into a baseball glove. She grinned. She had selected her mitt–with the trade name, "The Thief." I went to the mitts and tried several on, tossed a ball up and down. The anxiety shifted. I now felt disconnected, slightly disassociated from my body as though I was living behind myself, peering over my own shoulder. I kept having the impulse, which I resisted because I didn't want M. to think less of me, to make light of what I was doing. I wanted to laugh, to let the male clerk know that I knew that I was being silly. I wanted to act like a "girl."*

Alice Miller (1981), focusing on early childhood, observes that when children learn to censor their thoughts and feelings in order to be good, they lose or repress a part of themselves. "From the reconstructions available through analyses," she notes, "I have gained the impression that there are children who have not been free to experience the very earliest feelings, such as discontent, anger, rage, pain, even hunger and, of course, enjoyment of their own bodies" (p. 46). The prohibition against the free play of feelings results in a disconnection from feeling and from their bodies. By reconstructing themselves to fit ideals of goodness and perfection, these children create a self that functions so well that the underlying loss is often not evident except symptomatically, for example, in depression. Miller also explains that when parents, themselves too often disconnected from their desires and feelings by the requirements they have had to meet, attempt to do "the opposite" with their children than was done with themselves, they end up unintentionally repeating both the disconnection and pain of their lives in their children's–lives. Only if parents re-integrate their lost feelings and embody a different way of being, suggests Miller, can change occur between generations.

What does this mean for adolescent girls when "the enjoyment of their bodies" would involve playing with their sexuality? Passionate feeling and sexuality are lost to those who cloak themselves in conventions of feminine goodness; yet, if what Miller observes is true, these feelings will not just disappear: they will inhabit the body, creating profound dis-ease.

> *Suddenly, in my mind's eye, I could see my body from behind: down the calf of my right leg was a black lightning bolt. I had an immediate recognition of death and of the varicose vein in my right leg. My heart began to pound.*

If two recent studies of depression and other psychiatric disorders in high school students can be believed, girls in adolescence experience deep dis-ease in and with their bodies. These studies indicate that girls are experiencing depression twice as frequently as boys (Allgood-Merten, Lewinsohn & Hops, 1990; Whitaker et al., 1990). Girls' bodies, the Allgood-Merten study reports, are a source of acute distress for them. Yet, it is not their bodies, but their ideas of their bodies–what they should look like, what is attractive – that cause them such pain. As Julie, a reader of *Sassy* magazine (1990), wondered in a letter to the editors:

> When I got my August issue, I read in "Body Talk" that more girls get depressed than guys and the main reason is many (I suppose, myself included) are overly obsessed with their bodies, even though they may be perfectly normal for their age and height. Well, excuse me, but didn't "The And-You-Thought-You-Knew-the-Difference-Btween-Guys-and-Girls-Poll" in the same issue say that guys rated "looks" as their number-one priority in a girlfriend?! So I was thinking, maybe there's a little bit more to girls' obsessions with their bodies than just plain female neurosis.

Julie says, excuse me, but if boys are judging girls by their looks, then doesn't it make sense for girls to be "overly obsessed" by how they look? Moreover, she seems to ask psychologists how girls' discomfort with their bodies can be dismissed as neurotic when girls need to play up to boys and men? Julie seems to find it perfectly understandable that this would be depressing to girls. Yet, following Miller's logic, girls' depression might have underlying causes that Julie might not find immediately understandable: anger at being reconstructed as "looks" and losing the pleasure in one's now sexualized body.

> *My mother and I have varicose veins. She has them in both legs, as did her mother. I have them in my right leg. Whenever I would catch a glimpse of the rippling purple vein at the surface of my skin, I would get slightly nauseous. My mother warned me throughout high school that I was destined for varicose veins since all of the women in her family had them. I should take care, not stand on my feet too long, not go without support hose. She complained about the pains in her legs– the throbbing in her veins that happened when she was on her feet. I remember once she pressed her finger into my bulging purple vein and exclaimed, "When you get pregnant that thing is going to explode!" I nearly threw up. My legs, too, would*

> *throb when I stood for too long and were the first part of my body to tire. I waitressed summers through college wearing a polyester uniform and elastic stockings in 90 degree heat. Anything related to that vein made me queasy.*

Anorexics, the psychological daughters of Freud's hysterics, speak their dis-ease with their bodies. Susan Bordo (1989), in her reading of the "text" of anorexia, exposes the dazzling logic of femininity-gone-mad. Through the writing of anorexic girls, she describes the anorexic triumphing over desire for food:

> In the process, a new realm of meanings is discovered, a range of values and possibilities that western culture has traditionally coded as 'male' and rarely made available to women: An ethic and aesthetic of self-mastery and self-transcendence, expertise, and power over others through the example of superior will and control. (p. 23)

Bordo makes the connection between the adoption of these "male" values and success with an attempt on the girls' part to transform themselves by erasing the curves of their bodies to align with a culture that demands from them both traditionally male achievement and passive feminine perfection. In so doing, the girls solve the problem of the danger of being embodied as a woman. These girls quell their bodies' hunger for food and for sex: They reconstruct their desire as they disfigure themselves. This final solution allows them to enter the male world while maintaining the pristine virginity of childhood.

Catherine Steiner-Adair (1990), also, observes these privileged girls struggling with the demands for competitive achievement and conventions of femininity. She finds that the girls who play along with and adopt the current conventions of the "Superwoman"–the perfect wife, mother and executive–are more likely to have trouble with their eating. It is as if the different bodies required by these demands–the unfeminine male body and the nonsexual female body–can be achieved by a young woman if she strips her body of womanly characteristics, becoming a man-woman and child-woman simultaneously.

The black lightning bolt down the back of my leg clutched at my mind. The image wouldn't let go of me as I struggled to stay centered in my body by feeling my breath enter and leave me. I made my purchases as though I was a newscaster reading the agricultural report of an obscure foreign capital. While it made perfect sense for my vein and a death symbol to be related, I couldn't make some crucial connection. I kept trying to figure it out, wondering it over and over in my mind. I thought that part of the message was that I would die if I kept doing what I was doing. But that didn't have the resonance of true revelation. How am I going to die? I kept asking myself. Why? Suddenly, the lightning struck home: I wouldn't actually die but the self who thought she had to be certain ways in order to be my mother's daughter would die if I inhabited my body with the freedom that I had when I was 11, if I played with my father as my brothers did. The image vanished.

The madonna with her child (born without sex) expresses so beautifully the highest ideal of conventional femininity and human empathy. She sits serenely, her one breast exposed as the male child who will save humanity suckles. One hand is raised, palm out and open. The breast, in all of its sacred and profane incarnations, from the madonna to the air-brushed Playboy centerfold, signifies femininity. Odd – or perhaps not – that, figuratively speaking, it is the mothers of anorexic girls, that is, middle-to upper-middle-class white women, who have higher rates of breast cancer than any other group of women in this country (Levy & Wise, 1988).

As the image vanished, so did my queasy relationship with my varicose vein. I can look at it, touch it, wonder at its hideous progress. I've become an avid biker and swimmer. And my legs don't tire in the same way.

Freud (1905/1975), father of psychotherapy, viewed as normal the disconnection of adolescent girls' sexual desire from their knowledge. Increased repression in girls–a repression, in part, of all desire and particularly sexual desire–is thought to be ideally feminine. When the construction of "goodness" for women means ignorance of sexual arousal, and access to power–or, simply, survival–for women requires their bodies to be open to the gaze and grasp of men's attention, this repression should be expected, but hardly normal.

Yet, the vitality of women's sexual feelings resists being shut away in some underground cavern of psychic experience. According to Kinsey, Pomeroy, Martin and Gebhard (1953), most men reported masturbating to climax for the first time between the ages of 13 and 15 while women report masturbating for the first time (and often not to orgasm) at 25, 30 or 35. Kaplan and Sager (1971) compared the patterns of sexual activity among men and women and found that, while men have the capacity for intense genital response in late adolescence, this capacity develops in women around the ages of 35 to 40. A heightened capacity for intense sexual response in women in the middle of their lives suggests a reclaiming of a vital relationship with the body, perhaps a recapturing of an earlier playfulness.

"The hallmarks of loss," says Carol Gilligan (1990), "are idealization and [denigration, and under that–rage], and under the rage, immense sadness" (p. 511). Within a culture where girls' safety is so compromised by sexuality, some girls construct within themselves a logical compromise. The ideals that they take in and hold in their minds–ideals reflecting the construct of femininity–split their feelings for hunger, passion and play from their knowing. The result of this is a series of losses that live in the psyche, caught and frozen at the age where they were severed from consciousness. The transformation of the playing girl's body to the restrained woman's body marks a transition from mother's home to the man's world. The mother, friend of childhood and exemplar of womanhood, stands as a guide from the one body to the next. When she protectively warns her daughter of the dangers of desire in a violent androcentric culture–warnings that resonate loudly in countless images and ideas–the mother may unwittingly participate in her daughter's dis-ease with her body. The seemingly mysterious loss of connection with their mothers that some girls experience–the loss of a world of shared experience, touch, simple pleasure and anger - creates another gulf in the girl's psyche. The daughter is left doubly divided: from her own feelings and from comfort and connection with her mother. Rage–deep, inchoate, and forbidden to the ideal woman–fills the chasms dividing the self from herself and from the mother she loved and lost.

Yet, there is some play in this cycle. Mothers can guide their daughters to a different body: a playful woman's body. Acknowledging sexual desire as a source of erotic power and emotional knowledge is critical to the free play of feeling in the woman's body. To guide daughters to be responsible to and in their bodies, women need to free the erotic in themselves, to recognize the joy of the erotic in their daughters. The bloom of sexual intensity in women in middle adulthood could be a move by the psyche toward integration of body and idea, of the girl within and the woman one has become. Or, women may, as I have begun to do, retrace the path of the loss of the girl within by exploring her world of play. Playing with this girl brings back the conflict at the crossroads, and, perhaps, a reunion from which a new journey might begin.

REFERENCES

Allgood-Merten, B., Lewinsohn, P., & Hops, H. (1990). Sex differences and adolescent depression. *Journal of Abnormnal Psychology, 99*(1), 55-63.

Bordo, S. (1989). The body and the reproduction of femininity: A feminist appropriation of Foucault. In A. Jaggar & S. Bordo (Eds.), *Gender/body/ knowledge: Feminist reconstructions of being and knowing* (pp. 13-33). New Brunswick, NJ: Rutgers University Press.

Brown, L. (1989). *Narratives of relationship: The development of a care voice in girls ages 7 to 16.* Unpublished doctoral dissertation, Harvard University.

Duras, M. (1986). *The lover.* (B. Bray, Trans.). New York: Harper & Row.

Freud, S. (1895/1955). Fraulein Elisabeth von R. In J. Strachey (Ed.), *The standard edition: Studies on hysteria, Vol. II* (pp. 135-181). London: The Hogarth Press.

Freud, S. (1905/1975). The transformations of puberty. In J. Strachey (Ed.), *The standard edition: Three essays on the theory of sexuality Vol. VII* (pp. 66-88). London: The Hogarth Press.

Gilligan, C. (1990). Joining the resistance: Psychology, politics, girls and women. *The Michigan Quarterly Review, 29*(4), 501-536.

Kagan, J. (1972). A conception of early adolescence. In J. Kagan & R. Coles (Eds.), *Twelve to sixteen: Early adolescence* (pp. 90-105). New York: Norton.

Kaplan, H., & Sager, J. (1971). Sexual patterns at different ages. *Medical Aspects of Human Sexuality,* June, pp. 10-23.

Kincaid, J. (1985a). *Annie John.* New York: New American Library.

Kincaid, J. (1985b). *At the bottom of the river.* New York: Random House.

Kinsey, A., Pomeroy, W., Martin, C., & Gebhard, P. (1953). *Sexual behavior in the human female.* Philadelphia, PA: W.B. Saunders & Co.
Levy, S.M., & Wise, B.D. (1988). Psychosocial risk factors and cancer progression. In C.L. Cooper (Ed.), *Stress and breast cancer* (pp. 77-96). New York: John Wiley & Sons.
Miller, A. (1981). *The drama of the gifted child.* New York: Basic Books, Inc.
Say what [Letters to the editor]. (October, 1990). *Sassy Magazine.* p. 12.
Steiner-Adair, C. (1990). The body politic: Normal female adolescent development and the development of eating disorders. In C. Gilligan, N. Lyons, & T. Hanmer (Eds.), *Making connections: The relational worlds of adolescent girls at the Emma Willard School* (pp. 162-182). Cambridge, MA: Harvard University Press.
Suleiman, S.R. (Ed.) (1986). *The female body in western culture.* Cambridge, MA: Harvard University Press.
Tan, A. (1989). *The Joy Luck Club.* New York: Ivy Books.
Whitaker, A., Johnson, J., Shaffer, D., Rapoport, J., Kalikow, K., Walsh, B. T., Davies, M., Braiman, S., & Dolinsky, A. (1990). Uncommon troubles in young people: Prevalence estimates of selected psychiatric disorders in a nonreferred adolescent population. *Archives of General Psychiatry, 47*, 487-496.

Coming Out Against All Odds: Resistance in the Life of a Young Lesbian

Beth Zemsky

> With whom do you believe your lot is cast?
> From where does your strength come?
>
> (Rich, 1983, p. 12)

I remember the day I first met Maggie. I happened to be at the reception desk of the agency at which I worked, a family service agency that has a gay and lesbian counseling program, when Maggie called requesting an appointment as soon as possible. All I learned about her at the time was that she was lesbian and that she and her lover had been among a handful of protesters who had been hit by the police during a recent demonstration protesting then President Reagan's decision to send troops into Honduras. On the phone she sounded shaken but very clear and intentional.

During our first session, with the same clarity and intentionality, Maggie described the protest, her behavior, the behavior of the police, and the conflict which followed in which she perceived that the police had used excessive force. Maggie was scared and in pain, in part because she was hit in an area of her body where she had had a number of surgeries. However, Maggie was primarily angry. She

---

Beth Zemsky, MAEd, LICSW, is a community organizer and psychotherapist. She is currently Training and Consultation Coordinator for the Gay and Lesbian Community Action Council, Minneapolis. Ms. Zemsky wishes to thank Maggie, the Lesbian and Gay Counseling Program of Family and Children's Service of Greater Minneapolis, Elissa Raffa, and T.C. Largaespada for their support of this work.

firmly believed that the police had behaved unfairly – that yes, she had broken a trespassing law, but the officers' response had been disrespectful to the protesters and insensitive to the needs of the Honduran and Nicaraguan people. On the other hand, Maggie was also scared about her anger. She was concerned about the intensity of it and was worried that it might "come out sideways in [her] relationships." I remember thinking about the complexity and the passion of Maggie's personal and political stances even in the face of bodily injury and possible criminal charges. I knew Maggie was young, but I was surprised when I learned that she had just turned eighteen. I was grateful that the agency had a sliding fee scale that permitted me to charge Maggie just $5 an hour for therapy, so that we could begin our work together.

This first session began a relationship that continued for over two and a half years. During this time, Maggie learned about herself, her relationships, and the world in which she lives, while solidifying her identity and her ability to speak about what she knows. And I in turn learned a tremendous amount from her about ways a young lesbian can, with resiliency, creativity, and courage, resist others' expectations of her, explore who she is, name herself, and come out against all the odds of her doing so. In a culture that silences women and attempts, through pervasive sexism, homophobia, heterosexism,[1] and ageism, to render invisible young lesbian lives, I think that Maggie's struggle to claim an authentic identity during her late adolescence is a process worth examining.

How did Maggie manage these tasks during a developmental period that Gilligan (1988a) has described as the time when "thinking becomes self-consciously interpretive" and the "schemes of the culture, including the system of social norms, values, and roles, impinge more directly on perception and judgment, defining within the framework of a given society what is the 'right way' to see and to feel and to think?" (p. xxiii). How did she cope with the pressure towards conventionality in adolescence which, while problematic for all young women who are attempting to resist the cultural requirement to ascribe to traditional female sex roles, is intensified for a young lesbian who is struggling to claim "an identity they taught me to despise?" (Cliff, 1980).

In the following discussion, I will begin to respond to these questions first with a brief overview of relevant information and theory pertaining to the construction of a lesbian identity in a homophobic culture. I will discuss the ways in which Maggie maintained her resistance to the pressure to conform underground until it was "safe" enough to voice, and then how her search for a community affected her ability to voice her resistance by coming out. I will also examine Maggie's struggle to continue to express connectedness, even in the face of family, peer, and societal rejection, through her insistent search for continuing connections, and for solutions that included both herself and others. Finally, I will explore the need for lesbian adolescents to maintain continual resistance to preserve a uniquely "queer" voice, despite insistent cultural pressures to conform.

CONSTRUCTION OF A LESBIAN IDENTITY

According to epidemiological studies, it is estimated that 10 to 15 percent of the population is likely to be predominantly homosexual (Kinsey et al., 1953; Bell & Weinberg, 1978; Kinsey, Pomeroy, Martin, & Gebhard, 1953; Kinsey, Pomeroy, & Martin, 1948). The recent unprecedented growth of visible gay and lesbian communities in many parts of the country has created radically new possibilities for men and women to "come out" and give voice to their desire to live a particular lifestyle (Herdt, 1989). The visibility of these communities has also enabled younger women to have some role models and vague signposts pointing to possibilities in their process of identity acquisition.

"Coming out" can be defined as the process of recognizing one's sexual identity and integrating this knowledge into one's lifestyle (deMonteflores & Schultz, 1978). While the etiology of homosexuality (and of all sexual orientations) is unclear, both research reports and clinical interviews reveal that most persons who identify as lesbian had some internal awareness of being different in early childhood (Troiden, 1989). In these retrospective reports, most often women do not attribute this sense of differentness to lesbianism. Rather, they describe feeling different as a sense of "having an itch one can't scratch," of never fitting in and not knowing why, of being hidden underground. Women report carrying this vague knowledge of their differentness into adolescence, and sometimes beyond, without having a name for it and thus without a voice to express this knowledge or its implications.

Studies have indicated that the mean age for women to recognize and to pronounce (at least to themselves) that this sense of differentness and disquiet has something to do with lesbianism is approximately age fourteen (American Psychological Association, 1977; Gay and Lesbian Community Action Council, 1990). This acknowledgment is typically the outcome of a lengthy internal process that Cass (1979) describes as a search for interpersonal congruency.

According to Cass (1979), identity synthesis, the theoretical end point of the coming out journey, is a process of reconciling three aspects of self to the point to which they are internally congruent and express a coherent sense of identity to self and others. These three aspects are: (1) one's own self perception; (2) one's behavior; and (3) one's perception of others' view of self. These three aspects can be expressed in the following corresponding questions: Who am I? Does my behavior reflect who I perceive myself to be? Do I believe others perceive me in the same way I perceive myself?

The coming out process begins at the point at which the answers to any of these questions are incongruent with the answers to the others. For instance, a girl may be dating boys but perceive herself to be "not heterosexual." Or a girl could have a "special friend" whom she loves and with whom she is having sex and be perceived by others as heterosexual. Or, conversely, a girl could be labelled "butch" and "queer" due to her lack of adherence to the prescription for stereotypic feminine behavior whether or not she identifies herself as lesbian. All of these scenarios would create internal dissonance which would serve to push and pull a girl along internally in a process to reconcile the inconsistencies.

However, resolving these inconsistencies may necessitate defining oneself as different than one's family and peers. As Gilligan (1990) has noted, what is at stake for girls in adolescence is "the need to find ways of making connection in the face of difference" (p. 10). For a young woman coming out, this struggle is magnified. If she can resist the pressures of sexism and heterosexism, the young woman who is lesbian may have a chance of finding her own voice.

To develop interpersonal congrueney and to come out in a cultural atmosphere of homophobia and heterosexism presents a dilemma. How does a young woman stay connected to her knowledge that she is lesbian when this knowledge means risking rejection and isolation from family, peers, church, and the dominant culture? Until she has the psychological and relational resources to face these real risks, her survival may necessitate going underground, keeping her new knowledge about herself out of the public world.

MAINTAINING RESISTANCE UNDERGROUND

> I refuse to become a seeker for cures.
> Everything that has ever
> helped me has come through what already
> lay stored in me. Old things, diffuse, unnamed, lie strong
> across my heart.
> This is from where
> my strength comes, even when I miss my strength
> even when it turns on me
> like a violent master.
>
> (Rich, 1983, p. 10)

Maggie is the youngest child, and only daughter, in a caucasian, Catholic, white-collar working class family who live in a midwestern city. Maggie had three older brothers, one of whom died of an illness as a toddler shortly before Maggie was born. The death of this sibling, as well as some other situational factors, contributed to an atmosphere of high stress and little emotional engagement during Maggie's earliest years. Other than times when Maggie was being verbally reprimanded or physically disciplined for some real or imagined infraction of what seemed to her to be constantly shifting family rules, Maggie reports feeling invisible to her parents. This sense of invisibility included Maggie's perception that her parents did not attend to or protect her from the physical abuse she received from an older brother. She has stated that "I felt not welcome, like I wasn't supposed to be there. I wasn't supposed to cause waves or draw attention to myself. It was scary. I felt like a ghost. No one gave a shit if I existed. I was extra, dispensable."

As a child, Maggie coped with the stress and danger of her family situation by being "as good as possible" as a way to win approval, to gain some hope for positive attention from her parents, and to avoid negative consequences. She was a good student, involved in school, and was thought of by her teachers and peers as bright, personable and kind. She was also extremely self-sufficient. She learned to be able to attend to most of her physical needs, and the emotional needs she could recognize, without much parental assistance.

Another way that Maggie coped with the disengagement in her nuclear family was to search for a sense of connectedness with others within her young world. Key among these connections was her relationship with her grandmother, who lived on a farm not far from Maggie's family home. Maggie has described her grandmother and the farm to be a "pocket of caring" and "a place to be myself." Also Maggie found similar pockets of caring by "adopting the surrogate families" of her school friends. These other families, where she often spent mealtimes and weekends, provided places where she had different experiences of herself in relationship than she could have had at that point in time within her own family. Maggie's self-sufficiency and her insistent search for a sense of connection, both survival strategies she developed while quite young, would prove to be useful to her later on.

Until the age of eleven, Maggie appeared outwardly to be doing quite well, and she was not overtly distinguishable from the other girls who were her peers. However, she has described always internally "feeling this sense of being different, of knowing I was growing up hard, of feeling freakish." This sense of being different pushed her to try to fit in at school and with her peers and yet at the same time left her with a sense of despair about "not being ever right enough or perfect enough to do it [fit in] . . . of being alone." At the time, it was unclear to Maggie what this sense of differentness was about. She just knew that she felt different and that this felt "hard and confusing."

When Maggie was twelve, she began developing the first symptoms of what was to become a severe rare digestive tract disorder which is believed to be in part induced and exacerbated by stress. At first she tried to hide her worsening symptoms and her increasing physical pain from her family and friends by relying on her well learned self-sufficiency. She tried modifying her behavior, changing her diet, and cleaning up soiled clothes and bedding without anyone finding out. Despite these efforts, Maggie's illness challenged her strategy of self-sufficiency, which by this point had rendered her invisible and isolated in her physical suffering. Her illness forced her to reach out to her family for help. When Maggie's symptoms eventually got too difficult for her to manage, she finally told her parents and was hospitalized.

Despite her pain and her fear about her physical condition, Maggie describes that first hospitalization when she was twelve as one of the happiest times of this period of her childhood. During the weeks Maggie spent in the hospital, she had her parents' undivided nurturing attention for the first time she could remember. In addition, she had the nurturing attention of a caring and committed hospital staff around the clock. Maggie remembers eagerly awaiting being released from the hospital with the belief that the new connectedness in her relationship with her parents would continue. Even if she had an ileostomy, had missed a lot of school, and now had to take special medicines with every meal, returning home to be nurtured and taken care of by her parents "almost seemed worth it."

However, Maggie's newly discovered experience of her illness as a source of connectedness to her family did not last for very long. When she returned home, she found herself again needing to fend for herself but now with more and more pressing physical needs. She recalls feeling scared, but also relieved, when she discovered that she was to return to the hospital for a second surgery. "I didn't want another surgery, but I was glad to be going back to the hospital. I hoped things would be back with my parents there like they were the first time, and I knew no matter what that the nurses would take care of me." The hospital had become another "pocket of caring." Her approach to dealing with her illness had become a dangerous resistance strategy, a way of maintaining connections at a terrible physical cost.

Yet Maggie's approach to dealing with her illness was also rooted in a vital and healthy need for real connections. Maggie has described her illness "as a savior." Although she did not perceive her parents to ever again respond with the same quality of unconditional nurturing that they had shared during her first hospitalization, her illness did shift her relationship with her parents, and so with herself, in significant ways. Her illness challenged Maggie's strategy of unobtrusively living in an environment in which she was, for the most part, invisible and voiceless. Maggie had survived by being self-sufficient, "a good kid," and by searching for pockets of connection with others while working towards and hoping for a nurturing connection with her parents. Her illness challenged her ability to be completely self-sufficient, as she could no longer manage to meet her needs on her own anymore. Secondly, because Maggie had missed a lot of school and felt even more different from her peers due to her illness, she was no longer able to "hide out behind being so good anymore." Lastly, her experiences in the hospital reinforced and strengthened her search for connectedness with people outside of her nuclear family and, in this way, opened up new possibilities for nurturance. At this point in her development, at the age of thirteen, Maggie could "resist" her invisibility and her silence only through her illness. However, this psychological struggle, fought out on the battleground of her body, incurred a number of psychic and physical risks.

Maggie's illness presented the risk that she would be drawn to the attention and nurturing that she received from medical personnel and "take on the patient role" as a way to be connected and to belong. Unfortunately for Maggie, as for other women coping with disabilities, a path of searching for voice through connectedness with monolithic medical institutions as a survival strategy when all else seemed to have failed would have left her, in the long run, as invisible and voiceless as she had been in her family. It was with this backdrop of the increasing inadequacy of her existing modes of survival, and her fear "of becoming a chronically sick person, of being thought of as a gimp," that Maggie began her coming out process.

COMING OUT AS AN ACT OF RESISTANCE AND THE SEARCH FOR COMMUNITY

> That's why I want to speak to you now. To say: no person, trying to take responsibility for her identity, should have to be so alone. There must be those among whom we can sit down and weep, and still be counted as warriors . . . I think you

> thought there was no such place for you, and perhaps there was none then, and perhaps there is none now; but we will have to make it, we who want an end to suffering, who want to change the laws of history, if we are not to give ourselves away. (Rich, 1983, p. 33)

When Maggie was fourteen, she met a new friend, Kim, at school. This new friendship helped Maggie deal with some of the loss and isolation that had intensified since the beginning of her illness. Maggie described Kim as unlike anyone she had ever met before. She had different ideas, different cultural tastes and different views about how the world was organized. All of these differences were startling and very attractive to Maggie, as was Kim. The two girls quickly fell in love and more slowly began to experiment with each other sexually. For Maggie, her connection to Kim felt like a lifeline, a place where she was heard and seen both emotionally and psychically, where she no longer felt sick or invisible, or as drastically different as she had from her other peers. Being with Kim "felt right," even though their sexual contact challenged Maggie's beliefs about sexuality internalized from her family and her Catholic upbringing. Being with Kim "felt like coming home" to a sense of herself she had not known was possible. Maggie's "resistance" to invisibility and silence had taken a new turn; she experienced pleasure in her body and found a way to connect with another person that was not associated with pain and illness.

Maggie's relationship with Kim was a focal point for Maggie's life for almost a year, despite the increasing severity of her illness. Maggie did not yet define herself as lesbian during this time. She knew that she loved Kim, wanted to be with her and liked how she felt about herself in connection to Kim. She thought of Kim as "special," as this one girl she could feel this way about. According to deMonteflores and Schultz (1978), employing a "special case" scenario, that is, "I am not a lesbian; I just happen to be in love with this particular girl," is a common beginning point for many young lesbians. For Maggie, this stance created some internal dissonance that she was able quietly and discreetly to manage until Kim left their relationship when Maggie was 15. This leaving created another crisis.

> After Kim left, I was just depressed. I was home a lot with my family again, and alone. I had missed so much school, because I was sick, and I didn't care anymore . . . My teachers were all concerned, as were my parents. I would promise to do assignments by a certain day and then just not do them. This wasn't like me. . . They would say I was too bright to waste my talents, that I owed it to someone to make something of myself . . . I just knew that too much had happened, and I was different. The school stuff didn't matter in the same way anymore.

Kim's departure pushed and pulled Maggie to seek new ways to define herself. Other than "being good," which now meant denying some very powerful feelings and knowledge about herself that she had learned while with Kim, Maggie's family and school provided Maggie with no other models that would assist her in resolving her dissonance. As she had done so many times before, Maggie looked for other pockets of nurturing to support her in this process.

Most essential for Maggie during this period was her connection with a community-based gay and lesbian youth group. It was through her involvement in this group that Maggie began to be able to acknowledge something that she had known for a long time, "that I was different, that I was a lesbian, that I was queer, but it was okay and I wasn't alone."

Maggie's attendance at this group, her friendships with other group members, plus Maggie's worsening school record, led to a lot of conflict between Maggie and her parents. Her parents attempted to resolve this conflict by banning Maggie from the group and her new friends, whom they knew to be lesbian. Losing the group and her friends, losing this environment in which she had been able to voice who she was and what she knew about herself, again plunged Maggie into a depression and into a deep dilemma. How could she honor her parents' limits and be who they wanted her to be when to do so could mean losing the knowledge of herself and the voice she had just gained? How could she not abide by her parents' wishes when this could mean losing connection with them and possibly losing her home?

Maggie's response to the external conflicts and her internal turmoil was to leave her parents' home in an attempt to maintain her voice. At first she stayed with friends and then later in a placement with one of the adult lesbian leaders of the youth group with her parents' consent. As Maggie has stated, "Once I really knew that I was a lesbian, a queer, an absolute outsider, there didn't seem to be anything I could do anymore to fit what everybody wanted me to be. I would have had to totally give up me to do this." Although it was still a struggle, knowing she was lesbian made it easier for Maggie "not to get seduced into thinking if I just did x or y, everything would be okay. It didn't work when I was 'being good' or when I was sick, and it certainly wasn't going to work now." Coming out as a lesbian, stating who she was, provided Maggie with a means to acknowledge her voice. Her connection to a supportive gay and lesbian community gave her a way of maintaining a connection to this voice, despite the costs of and the pressures for silencing it.

THE SEARCH FOR INCLUSIVE SOLUTIONS

On the one hand, Maggie's coming out and her decision to leave her parents' home at age sixteen provided her with the opportunity to separate and move into the world independently with room to coiitinue to explore her voice. However, Maggie's separation from her family also accentuated a long-standing dilemma. How could Maggie be responsive to herself by coming out and yet, at the same time, preserve some connection with her family and all she had known, even if her family and culture had been so rejecting of her lesbianism? How could Maggie maintain a connection with her family without abandoning herself? Maggie chose to leave home at the point at which leaving was an alternative to silence in a situation in which her voice was squelched. But Maggie often wondered if it was "selfish to leave home" and "not to be there for them. What I was doing was hurting them." As Gilligan (1988b) has noted, "the option of exit leaves a problem of loyalty in its wake, a problem which if not addressed can lead to the decline of care and commitment in social relationships" (p. 146).

The conflicting loyalty for Maggie was the perceived opposition between a "selfish and selfless choice – an opposition where selfishness connotes the exclusion of others and selflessness the exclusion of self" (Gilligan, 1988b, p. 152). Despite her struggles with her family, leaving home and leaving her connection with her family behind as a way to resolve this dilemma was not a viable option for Maggie. Rather, she continued to try to find inclusive solutions in which she could both maintain a sense of herself and maintain a sense of connection with her family.

Specifically, Maggie's search for inclusive solutions included not only a continuing relationship with her family but also developing a diverse multi-generational network of friends in the lesbian community. This network of friends became Maggie's "family of choice" who could support Maggie's developing sense of congruency about her lesbian identity. With the solidification of her identity, she returned to the relationship with her family able to risk increased vulnerability in her attempts to make connections. These connections began with "safe topics of conversation" and expanded to include specific activities Maggie could do with her family that would both be an expression of herself and a bridge with family members. For example, Maggie planned carefully and intentionally to repair her car with her father in order to have a medium in which to connect to him. Consciously, she invited her parents to participate in her decision-making process about future educational plans. During one holiday season, she learned to perform songs that had been family favorites, so that she could share her love of music, something very important to her, with her family. What Maggie was attempting to accomplish with these efforts was to have a "real" connection with her family, one in which, as Maggie stated, "they are who they are and I am no longer invisible. I get to be me."

MAINTAINING CONTINUAL RESISTANCE

> I have wished I could rest among the beautiful and common weeds I can name, both here and in other tracts of the globe. But there is no finite knowing, no such rest. Innocent birds, deserts, morning-glories, point to choices, leading away from the familiar. When I speak of an end to suffering I don't mean anesthesia. I mean knowing the world, and my place in it, not in order to stare with bitterness or detachment, but as a power-

> ful and womanly series of choices: and here I write the words,
> in their fullness:
> powerful; womanly. (Rich, 1983, p. 35)

For Maggie and for other young lesbians, the need to maintain resistance in order to preserve voice does not end once a young woman has managed to declare herself to be lesbian. Research has indicated that coming out is a lengthy developmental process, with an average of 16 years from first recognition to identity synthesis (American Psychological Association, 1977). In addition, despite Maggie's successes in building a supportive community and bridging some of the gaps with her family, she continues to live in a world in which to be openly lesbian is typically met either with violence or silence. In 1989 alone, there were over 7000 cases of anti-gay related violence and hate crimes reported to a national gay anti-violence project (National Gay and Lesbian Task Force, 1989). In many legal and cultural settings, lesbianism is also still thought of as "the love that dare not speak its name" (Hall, 1928).

The pressure for Maggie to lose her lesbian voice and conform to heterosexual standards, in short to become invisible again, is a pervasive daily pressure. While Maggie feels proud of herself and proud of her lesbianism, "It is still not okay in the world for me to be okay." As another young lesbian group member stated, "We [lesbian youth] are thought of as dangerous, because we know who we are and we are not supposed to know. I hate when people tell me that it is okay for me to be lesbian, that it is not a big deal. Maybe they are personally accepting. This is good. But it is a big deal. Everyday it is a big deal. I don't like this being discounted."

For Maggie this pressure has necessitated adopting strategies of resistance into her lifestyle, which have included: ongoing involvement in community-based gay and lesbian youth support groups, choices of work and learning environments that would support her uniqueness (even if these choices lead to lower pay or less prestige), participation in radical political activities which reflect and support Maggie's desire to change the social structures that she perceives to be oppressive, and, given her ongoing health issues, choosing a health care practitioner who supports Maggie's wish to be in control of her body and her health care decisions.

REFLECTIONS

A survivor is:

> one who must bear witness for those who floundered; who tries to tell how and why it was they, also worthy of life, did not survive. And pass on ways of surviving; and tell our chancy luck, our special circumstances. (Olsen, 1979, p. 39)

While Maggie's means of maintaining her resistance, finding her voice and coming out are unique to her, there is much that I learned from working with her that informs my therapeutic work with other young lesbians. From our very first session, I developed a fundamental respect and trust for Maggie's abilities to survive and resist, capacities that preceded my involvement in her life. I translated that respect to Maggie through the stances and roles I took in our therapeutic relationship. For instance, despite a history that included abuse, a disabling illness, school problems, depression, leaving home at 16, and lesbianism, I did not view Maggie "as a troubled youth." I saw her as a survivor. A significant part of my role in our relationship was to learn from Maggie about the ways in which she had managed to resist. Specifically, I listened to Maggie speak about relationships and how they impacted her ability to resist and develop her own voice. I saw my job as helping her to acknowledge and learn about her own creativity, resiliency and strength and then getting and staying out of her way as she listened closely to herself.

It was also important that I be as present and clear as possible about my own voice in our therapeutic relationship. As a lesbian identified therapist, the simple fact that I had my own unique voice was an important model for Maggie. When I thought it was appropriate, I shared my thoughts, my opinions and my experiences. At times we discussed politics; at other times, psychological theory. I remained open to hearing Maggie's challenges, knowing that supporting her developing voice would on occasion even shake up the orthodoxy of the therapy itself. I accepted gifts she gave me, and, on the few occasions when we would cross paths at a lesbian community event, she would introduce me to her friends. It was important to Maggie that these parts of me be accessible to her as part of her search for inclusive solutions. And it was essential that my voice be clear and consistent in order to preserve the therapeutic boundaries that made these things possible and safe within the context of our connection.

During our last therapy session, Maggie stated, "I am realizing how much people make up my story and how precious is the way people weave in and out." We can learn much from the ability of young women, such as Maggie, to resist and name themselves against all odds. Our challenge as professionals is to remember this and listen.

NOTE

1. Homophobia is a complex prejudice defined as the irrational fear and hatred of lesbians, gay men and homosexuality in general (Weinberg, 1972). Homophobia is much like racism in terms of its xenophobic quality (i.e., it reflects a deepseated fear of people who are different and differentness in general). On another level, homophobia is a fear of one's own homoerotic (i.e., same sex sexual) feelings. Since, as Kinsey et al. (1948, 1953) revealed, approximately 50% of the general population have some same-sex sexual feelings, our cultural negativity about sexuality has led many to despise homoerotic sexuality despite its commonality. At a deeper level, homophobia is often expressed as a fear of violations of sex-role stereotypes. For instance, gay men are stereotypically perceived to be effeminate and female sex-role typed, while lesbians are thought to be "butch" and male sex-role typed. Conversely, anyone who acts in these cross-gender typed ways is thought to be gay or lesbian. In this way, this form of homophobia serves to keep all of us in line in terms of our sex roles in order to avoid being labelled "queer." Thus, homophobia serves to reinforce the entrenched sexism of our culture.

Homophobia, much like racism, sexism, anti-semitism, and classism, is institutionalized within our most basic social, religious, legal, and medical systems and is expressed as heterosexism. For instance, in most places in the country (with the exception of some local jurisdictions), lesbians and gay men do not have protection against discrimination in housing, employment, education, health care, child custody, etc. Furthermore, things such as the existence of sodomy statutes, the exclusionary practices of religious institutions, the often arbitrary and harassing response of the police and the courts, and the violent queerbashing backlash which has escalated since the beginning of the AIDS epidemic, all continue to convey the message to lesbians and gay men that our major institutions consider us to be criminal, sinful, sick and contagious persons.

REFERENCES

American Psychological Association's Board of Social and Ethical Responsibility (1977, November). Removing the stigma. *APA Monitor.*

Bell, A. P., & Weinberg, M. S. (1978). *Homosexualities: A study of diversity among men and women.* New York: Simon and Schuster.

Cass, V.C. (1979) Homosexual identity formation: A theoretical model. *Journal of Homosexuality, 4*, 219-235.

Cliff, M. (1980). *Claiming an identity they taught me to despise.* Watertown, Massachusetts: Persephone.

deMonteflores, C. & Schultz, S.J. (1978). Coming out: Similarities and differences for lesbians and gay men. *Journal of Social Issues, 34*(3), 59-72.

Gilligan, C. (1988a). Adolescent development reconsidered. In C. Gilligan, J.V. Ward, & J.M. Taylor (Eds.), *Mapping the moral domain.* Cambridge: Harvard University Press.

Gilligan, C. (1988b). Exit–voice dilemmas in adolescent development. In C. Gilligan, J.V. Ward, & J.M. Taylor (Eds.), *Mapping the moral domain.* Cambridge: Harvard University Press

Gilligan, C. (1990). Teaching Shakespeare's sister: Notes from the underground of female adolescence. In C. Gilligan, N.P. Lyons, T.J. Hanmer (Eds.) *Making connections: The relational worlds of adolescent girls at Emma Willard School.* Cambridge: Harvard University Press.

Gay and Lesbian Community Action Council (1990). *Northstar Project: Out and counted: A survey of the Twin Cities gay & lesbian community.* Minneapolis: Gay and Lesbian Community Action Council.

Hall, R. (1928). *The well of loneliness.* New York: Pocket Books.

Herdt, G. (1989). Introduction: Gay and lesbian youth, emergent identities, and cultural scenes at home and abroad. *Journal of Homosexuality, 17*(1/2), 1-42.

Kinsey, A., Pomeroy, W.B., & Martin, C.E. (1948). *Sexual behavior in the human male*. Philadelphia: W.B. Saunders.

Kinsey, A., Pomeroy, W.B., Martin, C.E., & Gebhard, P.H. (1953). *Sexual behavior in the human female.* Philadelphia: W.B. Saunders.

National Gay and Lesbian Task Force (1989). *Anti-gay violence, victimization, and defamation in 1989.* Washington, DC: National Gay and Lesbian Task Force.

Olsen, T. (1979). *Silences.* New York: Delta Dell Publishing.

Rich, A. (1983). *Source.* Woodside, California: Heyeck Press.

Troiden, R.R. (1989). The formation of homosexual identities. *Journal of Homosexuality, 17*(1/2), 43-73.

Weinberg, G. (1972). *Society and the healthy homosexual.* New York: St. Martin's.

“Do You Have Eyelashes?”

Hyo-Jung Kim

“Do you have eyelashes?” asked the little girl with blonde hair and blue eyes. I could only look at her momentarily, unable to meet her eyes as my face flushed deeply in shame. I was nine years old and had started a new elementary school. My parents had moved into a new house that they could call their own. The house became their symbol for success and reward for their patience and perseverance. For me, the move to the new house only meant moving to a new territory of landmines to traverse.

This is a story about my life as a Korean female growing up in the United States told in a series of vignettes. I was born in the Republic of Korea; in 1968, at the age of five, I moved from Korea to the United States with my family. As I tell this story, I speak about the ways that race, gender and culture shaped my own life, and by proxy, how they may affect the lives of other Asian-American girls and women. I believe this story is important for clinicians to hear, because so little has been written about Asian-American girls and women and the political and social contexts in which they live.

A STORY

“Flat face, flat face, that's not the only place!” “Chin, chong, chin, chong, ah-so!!” (The skin around the eyes pulled to the side.) “Yellow-face, can you see out of those eyes?!” Every day for nearly one year, I heard those words as I rode the bus to middle

---

Hyo-Jung Kim, MAR, EdM, is the Associate for the Feminist Liberation Theology Program in the Episcopal Divinity School, Cambridge, MA, USA. She is also Assistant to the AHANA (African, Hispanic, Asian, Native American) Coordinator at Simmons College Office of Admission.

school. I was eleven years old in seventh grade. A white boy had decided that it would be fun to ridicule me. He and two of his friends taunted me and humiliated me as others on the bus laughed at their jokes. Every day as I boarded the bus, I looked at white eyes that stared at me with spite and curiosity. For years, I could never talk about the humiliation, the sense of disgust and self-hate I had for myself. I must have done something to deserve such anger, I thought. I only understood the pain. This pain was familiar to me.

When I entered middle school the year before, I was ten years old. I was determined to do well in school and make my mother proud of me. I believed that speaking English well was the key to success in school. I sensed that to be a "true" American, I had to speak perfect English, to sound like a white person. In my determination to achieve this success, I believed that I had to remove any possible barriers. I decided that I would focus all my attention on learning English; I did not continue to learn Korean, the language which was spoken at home by my family. I began to resent my Koreanness, a resentment that was difficult to avoid in a culture that prizes English as the superior language.

Speaking Korean in an anglocentric, monolingual culture made me "other." I wanted to be like the other children in my class. I had learned in this country that to be different – from the standard of whiteness and maleness – to be other, meant to be inferior and bad. Everything about me was different. With the onset of puberty, my body began to change, and I did not want to change into something even more different from the other girls. Eyelash curlers would not make my eyes more round. They still appeared slanty and devious-looking. Perms made my hair wavy and pretty, I thought. I yearned in front of the mirror, wishing for a face that would save me from ridicule and shame. A white face would make others respect me, I wanted them to respect me. I knew that whiteness was part of what was required to have power in the United States.

To speak English fluently with a white, middle-class accent became my strategy for gaining respect from white people. Although I could not change my facial features, I could change the way I spoke the dominant culture's language. I endeavored to be a "true" American. Despite this decision, I continued to speak Korean minimally, since my mother spoke only Korean – her effort to retain her Korean identity and her children's. Throughout middle school, I was pleased with my new endeavor, which became more and more "successful." My grades were strong. I was convinced that I had made the right decision until the end of my eighth grade year, when it was time to select classes for high school. Confident of my academic abilities, I selected honor-level courses for science and mathematics. But my math teacher believed that I was too ambitious, and she instructed me not to take honors classes.

Devastated and ashamed, I accepted her evaluation of my academic abilities. Like my other teachers who awarded me with good grades, she did not encourage me to pursue further academic challenges. My efforts to convince my teachers that I was not stupid had failed. I spoke English like a US-born, white, middle-class person, and still I failed. In the end, I concluded that it did not matter how well I spoke English; my Korean face would be an academic liability. Ashamed and humiliated, I returned home that day to my mother, who was cooking food as she usually did when I returned from school. She listened as I told her what my teacher said. As she did so often, she encouraged me to take the honors math class, and she offered to help me with my homework. But I refused, believing that my teacher was right. It was a bitter lesson I learned that year in "the land of freedom and opportunity:" Hard work and initiative would not be rewarded and encouraged. The rules that I had learned so well did not apply to me. My Korean face and name would determine how others would treat me.

* * *

I entered the first grade when I was five years old. No one noticed that I was one year too young. I did not know a word of English. Unable to speak English, I spent the first two years of school in complete silence. I was not able to communicate with my teachers and classmates. I could not read the school textbooks or blackboard. Sitting in the classroom in silence, I began to learn a new culture and language. To this day, I still cannot remember those early years.

By third grade, I had learned to speak English. That year, I was placed in a special education class for slow learners. I was very confused about my placement in this class. For many years, I believed that I was stupid. I remember sitting in the class, asking myself why I was placed in this class. It was not until many years later, when I was in graduate school, that I realized I had been placed in that class because I spoke English with an accent and I was slow in understanding my teachers and the books that I read. My accent was the result of my speaking Korean at home, while I spoke English at school. To speak with any kind of accent was reason enough to be labelled stupid.

* * *

As each year passed, my sense of inferiority grew. I hated school. School was the unfamiliar culture of the dominant white society, while home was the familiar culture of Korean society. I lived in two cultures. I spoke two languages. I learned two sets of norms, value systems, and standards. I learned two different worldviews, two histories (see also Anzaldua, 1987). Through humiliation and scorn, I learned about my place in US society. I felt pride as a Korean whose culture had produced greatness and longevity, yet others were repelled by my Koreanness. I had to negotiate two dissociated cultures, living with two cultural frameworks in a society that values only one.

* * *

When I was in school, my mother did not speak English. Before she began working with my father in their variety store, she worked in a factory with other non-English speaking immigrant women. My father worked seven days a week, sixteen hours a day. Theirs was the "classic immigrant" story.

"Success" often comes at great cost. For my family, the cost, I believe, was too high. Years of struggle created great stress, depression, anger, frustration, and disappointment in my parents. Racism in the United States, even in a middle-class, "liberal" neighborhood, created a culture that made our lives invisible. We lived isolated, separated from others, because we were racially and culturally different. But who wanted to hear about the struggles of Asian immigrants? It seemed to us that white America wanted to hear only about the hard-working, good person who becomes a success story (see also Woo, 1983). To know about the actual details of the lives of Asian immigrants would mean that white people might have to begin to question the myth of the American dream. Of course, no one wanted to hear about our lives, our struggles to survive in a country that breeds racism and xenophobia.

My mother is a survivor; she survived Japan's brutal occupation of Korea, World War II, the division of Korea, and the Korean War. She was born into the Yangban (aristocrat) class in Korean society. Her family lost everything during the Japanese occupation. Forced to live as a stranger in her own country and to support the livelihood of foreigners, my mother learned to survive. Her language was banned from being spoken publicly. She was forced to take a Japanese name and to learn about Japanese superiority in school. Her culture and history were being systemically eliminated by the Japanese. Despite the threat of imprisonment and death, she and other Koreans continued to speak Korean. My mother understood racism and cultural genocide. She understood fear and intimidation. As a child, I listened to the stories of my mother's childhood. We were drawn together in our common experiences of oppression. I learned defiance and determination from my mother, my role model, my mother was a pillar of strength and hope. She had survived genocide and devastation, and I, her daughter, was convinced that I too could overcome all adversity. From her, I learned to be a survivor. Despite my mother's hopes that I would not have to struggle as she did, I did struggle.

To live with racism, sexism, and xenophobia was a lesson in daily survival. I learned that the United States was not my home. I felt like a stranger in a foreign land, always reminded by whites that I was not wanted. I lived with a daily silence that had been forced down my throat. In response to the daily violence of racism and sexism in my life, I took a combative stance, as I still do at times. Enclosed in an invisible shell that distilled the hate of racism, I prepared to engage in war as I marched off to school each day. In part, this preparation came from my mother, who had taught me to survive as she did. Knowing that the outside world was hostile and dangerous, my mother taught me to be proud to be Korean. My only means of survival was to do well in school and keep white people comfortable, so that they would not be angry with me. I used my invisibility in the classroom to stay alive.

However, to live in this way daily has its toll. To live under siege meant that my resistance was constantly vulnerable to corrosion. Over a period of time, I began to take on the image – an image that had been projected on me – to see myself as a passive, quiet Oriental girl, a "good girl" by white standards, but not good enough. I could not understand the hatred I felt around me; I only lived with this hatred.

* * *

On television, I saw movies with white people. White people killing savage red, brown, yellow, and black people. I don t remember seeing movies with Asian people with the exception of "The World of Suzie Wong," a movie about a Chinese female prostitute who falls in love with a white male military officer. Charlie Chan and Mr. Moto were played by white, European male actors who wore make-up to effect Asian eyes. Magazines displayed only white, blond, blue-eyed, tall, anemic women as the ones who were beautiful. Women of color were whores, maids, or worse, they did not exist in the movies, magazines, or television.

I saw the popular US television show, "M*A*S*H," which succeeded in bringing the Korean War into the national consciousness of the American public. I realize now that although the Korean War was nearly forgotten in US history books, "M*A*S*H" documented the War. However, the producers of "M*A*S*H" sacrificed Korean cultural accuracies to create an anti-Vietnam War statement. As a young girl at home, I learned about the Korean War through my mother who was sixteen when the War started. I understood what the war had done to Korea and her people, and what it had done to my family. I understood also what war does to those who stand on the other side of the aggression. I learned that the aggressors do not understand the real impact of war on the lives of people. I recall that the aggressors do not understand the real impact of war on the lives of people. I recall the day when a white boy eagerly asked me if I was North or South Korean. I was nine or ten years old. I protested that I was Korean, but he continued to press me until I told him that I was born in South Korea. At that moment, he was pleased that I was one of "the good guys," and he informed me proudly that his father had fought on the side of "the good guys." He walked away merrily, leaving me as I began to cry, because I had lost a grandmother and two uncles during the War. My mother is North Korean. From that day on, I vowed never to talk to an American about the Korean War.

Silenced by the dominant white culture, silenced by the white people, I was told who I was, what I was, and who I should be. Silenced by my school teachers who taught in a school that was eurocentric, monolingual and neo-colonialistic, I learned to live with the silences. I closed my mind to their thinking. I learned to regurgitate their words and their worldview. I learned to be a good student, reciting what my teachers wanted to hear. I chose to ignore white people when I heard condescension in their voices. School became a place where I learned the lessons of survival in a white racist culture: I learned to not make white people mad at me.

My seed of anger grew larger and larger. I grew to despise and distrust white people. Each venture out of my house became a journey into the darkness. Walking to school daily became a painful challenge for me. I grew to expect the classroom to be a frightening, humiliating place. The start of a new school year was often uncomfortable and frightening for me. Each year, I would have to endure the humiliation of hearing my name being mispronounced by teachers and being laughed at by my classmates. I dreamed of being somewhere else, disappearing into my chair. I dreamed of being free from the torment of school, an alien, threatening place.

In the face of disappointment and bitterness, I knew that I could not become or be an American, because I was not white. In my experience, an American was defined by skin color and ethnicity: whiteness and Western European. Perhaps my endeavor during middle school was my attempt to test the definition, to question the dominant culture's definition. With the failure of this endeavor, I embarked on a new path, a path towards self-understanding as a Korean female.

* * *

Fourteen years old, I rejected the ways of my white classmates, staying home on the weekends with my mother. I made a conscious effort to improve my Korean. Like a ghost, I existed in the school, always using my invisibility to survive. School, especially during middle school, had always been dangerous, but now I saw the danger as more than individuals threatening me. I began to see the danger as an institutional one. My brother came home one day from college and sat down and asked me if I was a feminist. I thought he was crazy, but I began to read the writings of Emma Goldman and Rosa Luxemburg. My path of resistance took the form of political awareness: I began to see sexism, to dissect and analyze the dominant culture, to know the histories of oppressed peoples in the United States, to know how people of color are pitted against each other economically, to understand that monolingualism serves to train young minds into seeing the world as either/or, to believe that there is only one reality, one history, one worldview, one way of speaking.

* * *

"I think that the success that you have achieved is a testimony to what can be accomplished in the United States," said my college roommate. We had so many arguments that ended with words like these. Typically, I would end our conversations, unable to make her understand my experiences.

"What are you complaining about? You have had it easy here. Imagine if you were living in Korea, your life would be miserable as a woman!" With those words, my friend rejected my experience as a Korean female living in the U.S. Shocked and surprised, I stopped talking to him. Years of sharing my experiences with him did not lead to any understanding on his part.

Near the end of college, I began to understand more than just the hate. I learned about breaking the silence, about speaking as an "I", not as an object of scorn and contempt. One day, I read *Sister Outsider* by Audre Lorde (1984). Lorde writes that "we were never meant to survive as human beings (p. 42)." These words forced me to notice the fear that I had and still live with. I had grown up afraid for my life. I read the words of a woman who understood my life finally. "For to survive in . . . america, we have had to learn this first and most vital lesson – that we were never meant to survive, not as human beings. And neither were most of you here today, black or not (p. 42)." For years I had remained fearful, always afraid of my visibility as an Asian female. To speak would be dangerous, I believed. I would be seen and I would be annihilated by white people. It seemed safer to remain silent, to use the silence as a shield.

* * *

I was not ready to begin to break the silence – to speak publicly about my experiences – until one day two years ago, when one of my nieces told me that her teacher did not like her and seemed to have singled her out for criticism. My other niece also told me about the times when kids called her "chink" and "chinese." She protested often by telling that she is Korean, but the black and white kids continued to tell her that "they" are all the same. I gave my nieces comfort, love and affirmation, wanting them to know that they are not deserving of such treatment. Indeed, they are not, nor was I. My silences have not protected them or me. The racial slurs, the hostile and curious stares, the dismissive attitudes of my teachers, the condescending tones in the voices of white adults. My teachers spoke to my white classmates with attention and interest, while I was spoken to with disinterest and boredom. White eyes looked through me as though I did not exist. White hands afraid to touch my hands as they place the change of money on the counter. Ignoring me as I stand in line for service, the white salesperson serves a white person who stood behind me. I became enraged, angry that things have not changed.

ON SPEAKING

"Whether we speak or not, we suffer" (Lorde, 1984, p. 42). In order to transform the silence into language and action, as Lorde writes, I had to face the terror within myself, the terror that kept me from speaking. Deep in the crevices of my mind, the place where my secret feelings are kept, I see the face of the child who is sad and crying. I see the face of the child who is me. To speak about my experiences is to speak about the dangers that have permeated my existence as a girl of color and then as a woman of color in the United States. I was not meant to survive with my body and mind as they are now. I was trained to believe in my inferiority, trained to believe that my purpose in life was to serve white people.

"Model minorities" have qualities the dominant culture values.

We possess light-colored skin, and we work hard without complaining. We are the "good" colored people. This myth of the model minority is an unyielding, impermeable one that white people do not want threatened. When I speak about my life as a Korean woman, white people begin to argue with me. They ignore me and they silence me. My words about racism, xenophobia, the economic exploitation of Asian immigrants, and cultural ignorance in the United States have no meanings, no coherence to those who believe the myth. White people often feel entitled to inform me about what I really mean when I say that I have experienced racism in my life. They tell me that they cannot believe that I actually live with racism because they don't see it and they like Asian culture. Dismissed with a gesture, I have been silenced. My words are unpleasant to the ears of white people, so therefore they no longer give me their attention. Once they are satisfied that they have made their point, they end the conversation with me.

To be angry means to be alive, to resist the oppression. To know that I was not treated with dignity or respect, to know that I was worthy of more from my teachers and classmates, in elementary, secondary, and higher education. To name the lies told in school, in the media, in the dominant culture. To break the silence means to speak the truths. To speak for yourself, no longer allowing others to distort your story. To name the racism means to debunk the myth of white, Euro-American, male superiority. When I speak, I am no longer an object. I become an active participant in the world. To speak means to have power, the power to name one's reality. The struggle to speak is the struggle against the racism, sexism, classism and xenophobia that destroys my people. When I speak my native language, I say that there is another reality, another way of living, another set of beliefs, another history that is real, thriving, and alive. I have begun the transformation of silence into language. To face the fear that keeps me from speaking means facing the dominant culture in which I live. I can no longer afford to remain silent about racism and the cultural genocide of my people. My nieces and unborn children cannot afford my silence. I must speak and speak now.

REFERENCES

Anzaldua, G. (1987). *Borderlands, La Frontera.* San Francisco: Spinsters/Aunt Lute.

Lorde, A. (1984). *Sister outsider.* New York: The Crossing Press.

Woo, M. (1983). Letter to Ma. In C. Moraga & G; Anzaldua, (Eds.), *This bridge called my back.* New York: The Kitchen Table Press.

SECTION IV: NOTES FROM THE UNDERGROUND

Adolescent Resistance and the Maladies of Women: Notes from the Underground

Teresa Bernardez

> A science of the life-world is interpretive and displays what is at play in the act of interpretation. Along with the phenomena reported, my presence as an investigator and reporter of findings is required. (Paget, 1990, p. 153)

THE CASE OF BETTY: A PROBLEMATIC PICTURE OF HEALTH

When I was a psychiatrist at The Menninger Foundation in 1962, I participated in the evaluation of data collected and analyzed by Dr. Lois B. Murphy, principal investigator of a longitudinal research

Teresa Bernardez, MD, is a training and supervising faculty at the Michigan Psychoanalytic Council and a former professor of psychiatry at Michigan State University, where she did her research on the cultural prohibitions governing the behavior of women.

project on Personality Development begun with Kansas infants and their families. By the time I joined the research team, the children subjects were in adolescence, and the data collected throughout the years was enormous. I was particularly interested in a number of girls who were of superior intelligence as children and who began to lose IQ points in adolescence, while becoming "appropriately feminine." Betty was one of those children. The description of Betty that follows is taken, with some minor changes, from a case report I wrote at the time:

> Betty was an energetic baby, vigorous, outgoing and alert. She developed into a very bright and capable youngster; the research record stated that she was "constitutionally sturdy, prone to activity, [a child] who finds delight in muscular movement, and who is well endowed in this area." From the very beginning, Betty defeated her mother's dream and expectation that she be a "feminine" daughter, meaning delicate, fragile and passive. Moreover, Betty grew up among boys; three younger brothers were added to the family when Betty was two, four and five years old. The boys and their games gave Betty an outlet for her expansivity, her active and exploring traits, her need for large muscular activity. Through her development during the preschool years, it was noticed by the researchers that her freedom of movement was not sacrificed to a feminine interest in her appearance, although some feminine interest did develop by the time Betty was four years old. Apparently, it gave Betty more pleasure to be the executor of her destiny as a vigorous person than to rejoice in being admired as a pretty object. She liked especially to fix things, to take things apart and put them together, as her father fixed things about the house.
>
> As she grew up and these traits became more evident, the mother's dislike of what she saw as a masculine side of Betty was more obvious. She made several comments to the research observers about her disappointment over the fact that Betty did not keep herself clean and that Betty preferred to be dressed in comfortable clothes if she was to play. These comments were frequent enough to suggest to the researchers that the girl

> perceived her mother's dissatisfaction. Betty was determined and hard to bend. Observers felt that her disobedience toward her mother was as conspicuous as that of her siblings: in Mrs. A's eyes, though, Betty was "the hardest to handle of her children."

Concurrent with a development towards more "feminine" behavior, the researchers reported that "Betty's Full Scale IQ was 12 points lower than in latency and [at early adolescence] 30 points lower than in preschool age." I noticed that Betty appeared to be adjusting to the demands of her environment by becoming "duller" in intelligence, more compliant and helpful to others; I was also aware of an absence in Betty of any development of "symptoms" of psychological distress. This picture was particularly gloomy to me at the time, because no one perceived Betty as troubled. The loss in her IQ points seemed to go unnoticed, since she was superficially happy and well adjusted. Dr. Murphy, who led the team, supported my concern and encouraged my inquiry into the factors that played a role in the loss of IQ in so gifted a girl. It was through my own relationship with Dr. Murphy that I read and reviewed for the Menninger Bulletin a crucial book for me at that time: The *Ferninlne Mystique* (Friedan, 1963). This book was the first eye-opener in my search for understanding about the fate of girls and the difficulties of women with and in our world.

THE KNOWLEDGE OF FEMALE OPPRESSION IN CLINICAL WORK WITH WOMEN AND GIRLS

I have been particularly struck by the research findings reported by Gilligan, Brown and Rogers (1990) revealing an undiscovered landscape of female adolescence, in which girls appear to have psychological difficulty coming into relationship with this culture. Their findings concord in important ways with my clinical experience with adolescent girls and with adult women. I think that understanding the experience of adolescent girls demands a perspective and sensitivity that calls attention to what is censored or unseen; the capacity to take on this perspective and sensitivity requires a preexistent knowledge and interpretation of the situation of women in this culture. Central to this endeavor is the importance of unearthing suppressed voices, which is the approach that Gilligan, Brown and Rogers (1990) take. I will outline three features of working with girls and women that I think are critical for researchers and clinicians engaging in this process.

1. Mutuality and responsiveness in interaction. I suggest that girls reaching adolescence, and women, are particularly sensitive and enabled by responsive and involved interactions rather than "objective" and impersonal attempts that might garner a more unspecific or indeed conventional response to queries about their lives.

2. The knowledge of women's experience in the social world and listening for healthy resistance. Researchers and clinicians working with girls and women need to have knowledge about the situation of women in the social world and to acknowledge and value that girls' and women live their lives as members of a large oppressed group. I find that having this awareness alters decisively my view of "symptoms" and of "resistance," which I will explain in the final section of this paper. This perspective calls for definitions of female psychological health in ways that authenticate female experience.

3. Listening with the third ear. The assumption made by psychoanalytic methods of interviewing is that a person discloses metaphorically or through associations a less conscious, more conflictual but quite meaningful set of communications; when a clinician hears properly and responds to them, the unveiling of a different set of data occurs. A main thrust of the work of Gilligan and her group has been to show the way in which women's and girls' voices have been made inaudible, because they do not fit traditional theories of development. Researchers and clinicians need to be alert to suppressed voices in order to share the knowledge that cannot be overtly spoken by girls and women within the constraints of this culture.

THE CASE OF MARITA: DEFIANCE AND HEALTHY RESISTANCE

Marita was brought to me by her mother when she was sixteen years old, because she was making her mother's life impossible.

She was skipping school, she was keeping all sorts of bad company – children with odd hairdos who had been abandoned by their parents, truants – and her behavior was erratic and difficult to control. Marita's mother was afraid that her daughter was on drugs and that Marita's sassy and angry behavior with her and with school authorities would bring her to the edge of expulsion. Her mother was also concerned that Marita would get pregnant and end up in a reformatory. And, in fact, I too thought that would be her fate when I first saw this impudent, lively, somewhat provocative youth, dressed to make heads turn.

Marita was angry, indeed, and demonstrated a great deal of concern for the down and out, but it was clear that she resented her mother's favoritism towards her brother, her insistence that Marita polish her ways to be able to get married, and her token concern about Marita's school failure. She was adamant about seeking adventure rather than playing it safe. She confessed that she did not care if she got pregnant and said that school was boring and was making "an idiot" out of her. Many of her complaints – if exaggerated – were based on reality and showed her intelligence, wit and sensitivity. Her posture of abandonment and love of risk barely hid a frightened, disappointed and lost youngster who was looking for shelter. Marita was defying me to reject her too, and I could see that she had already placed most of her bets on my abandonment.

My ability to identify with Marita served me well. My own adolescence had been full of fury and scorn. My efforts to defy the restrictions imposed blandly on women had been incoherent, but I had a similar frightened side, a similar aloneness. I took Marita seriously, and I expected her to respond to me in kind. She seemed to know that I was a survivor of similar battles, and she enjoyed my undisguised enjoyment of her, a thing so rare since she had been such a "bad girl!" Contrary to Marita's expectations, I revealed Marita's courage to her mother and helped her sympathize with Marita's struggles to have a life of her own, full of adventure and richness. In my attempt to make a different sense of her behavior to her mother, Marita was astonished to hear, for the first time, a different version of her story. She could not quite believe, but was struck, by my defense of the authentic pieces of valor and frankness that I saw in her behavior. I praised her intelligence and her humor, confessing that if she were older she probably would have a more responsive audience for her derisive criticism of her contemporaries. I was firm with her mother that it was very important to acknowledge the sense that Marita made of her social world and not to be carried away by her language, which tended to offend, because she had not succeeded in being heard in any other way.

Marita's story has tragic commonalities with the fate of other girls her age. She told me in secret that she had been sexually abused by her father since age 12, and that her father had threatened her with his suicide if she told her mother about it. He was furious and abandoned her when she refused his advances, and her school performance became the point of expression for Marita's secret drama. Against her teachers, the unreliable and uncaring authorities, she was contemptuous and defiant. Her anger and dislike of women was intense, and she felt they were all "patsies." Men were no better, but at least they offered her at this time the illusion of a romantic and adventurous life, empowerment through her sexual attractiveness and a refuge from a life without love and without a center. It was my acknowledgement of her anger in support of her dignity that led us to examine what she could best do with it. She had been defeating her purposes because she had realized them herself only dimly, and she was alone and without support. But once the painful search began, her anger would often turn to grief, to resurge again and again each time we connected it more and more clearly with abuses, deceptions, and betrayals. She could now articulate her complaints; she no longer allowed those around her to disregard them. When she could see, through her connection with me, how she was attached to the very people whom she distrusted, she could involve them rather than dismiss them.

The case of Marita is grave but not uncommon. This bright girl, who ended up receiving a scholarship for college, was the target of all the prejudices and inequalities that infuse the lives of women. Hers was an occult and shameful drama, but one which I have observed in other girls with similar histories of promiscuity, drugs and school truancy or poor performance. By working within a perspective that acknowledges the oppression of women in this culture, I have been able to discern, with Marita and with other adolescent girls, particular etiological factors which recur again and again:

grave disappointment about their fate as women, unequal treatment in relation to their brothers, history of sexual abuse and observing a devalued female in the household who allows herself and her daughter to be mistreated. Pressured to conform, disapproved of in her attempts to reject the false and hypocritical expectations of her family and society who neither could see her brilliance nor care about her exploitation and degradation, Marita was rebelling in ways that neither saved her from destitution nor got others to attend to and respect her plight. Interpreting Marita's defiance as healthy and worthy of support was fundamental to her recovery and optimal use of her abilities. The knowledge of female oppression and of women's difficulties in expressing their disappointment, conflict and anger with their circumstances in the world permits validation of the patient's experience of oppression and supports the emergence of a more authentic and resolute self.

IMPLICATIONS FOR THE TREATMENT OF WOMEN

The role played by the social demands made of girls by those around them to conform to the definitions of femininity, and the various ways in which these children feel abandoned by their mothers and others, is often absent in evaluations of these patients. Women's situation is not seen as an oppressive state, because this state of oppression has been defined by the group in dominance; it represents the status quo and therefore is accepted by all as a "norm" (Lugones, 1990). Ours is a society given to interpret as signs of "illness" the problems it generates in women who cannot quite fit into the small mold to which they are assigned. This habit of labelling as illness the discomfort which results from women's efforts to fit this crippling mold contributes to the oppression of women. The diagnosis of women who are resisting conformity as "ill" invites and substantiates more efforts to subdue these women into conforming through "treatment" of biological or psychological bent. Diagnosis and treatment in the cases of women who are unconsciously resisting conformity represent an acceptance of the status quo and indicate a blindness to the potential strength in the woman who is acknowledging and challenging a state of oppression.

I suggest that adult women have accomplished a profound burial of the discomforts of adolescence, such as those Marita suffered. Women who have "successfully" adapted to what the culture indicates is proper or desirable for women become inadvertent supporters and teachers of the status quo, since they demonstrate by their behavior that adhering to the norms of female behavior incurs no loss and accrues immediate and long term benefits. Our women patients, by definition, have not "succeeded" in adapting without symptoms. In many of them, the traces of their adolescent struggle can be perceived still, despite their attempts to disconnect and disconfirm these early ways of knowing the real problems they encounter in their situations as females in this culture.

The observations of Brown (1989) that in adolescence girls begin to aspire to be the "perfect girl," an impossible model of behavior that appears free from "unloving features," validates my own work on the social determinants of women's conflicts with anger (Bernardez, 1988). A central lesson that girls learn about being the "perfect girl" is that she does not get angry. This unlearning of a central feature of emotional life during adolescence that Brown has observed in girls emerges in adults in the portrayal of the "loving woman. One of the most critical associations with the adolescent part of themselves is women's denial of their anger, their fear of this unacceptable force that raises itself against the assiduous assaults that women encounter in daily living. I have found the damaging psychological effects of this cultural prohibition against the expression of anger on their own behalf again and again in adult women. The troublesome nature of the emotion of anger is already found in incipient form in the younger girls (Brown, 1989): Anger is an emotion that makes them vulnerable to criticism and isolation.

The consistency with which the girls in the work of Gilligan, Brown and Rogers (1990) and others speak of looking up to the perfect girl and becoming "good" by banishing all traces of unacceptable anger is very much in consonance with the pictures of psychological distress that many women present in their adult lives. For instance, in depression, a prevalent disorder of women, a woman's burying of her protest and unhappy submission to her fate may play a large role in producing her symptoms. In the evanescent disorder of premenstrual syndrome, "PMS," women vent their anger every month protected by the labeling of this disorder as one which affects women's "hormonal" balance; women's anger is thus justified and permitted, because it does not alter the status quo. In the so-called "Multiple Personality Disorders" so often found in victims of childhood sexual abuse, patients consistently dissociate their rage. The characters or "personalities" that carry the anger are predominantly male and thus can express this emotion without barriers. In women who suffer from agoraphobia, the consistent finding of excessive submission to a tyrannical and domineering husband in a caricature of "feminine" dependency is played out with a terror of expressing anger, which precedes panic attacks. All of these are prevalent disorders of women in our culture and at this time. In each of these diagnoses, women have further dissociated themselves from the label of "bad woman" (Lugones, 1990) by becoming "ill," which, ironically, enables them to remain faithful to the expectations of the dominant culture.

I suggest that as clinicians we can develop a growing awareness of how adolescent girls and women try to speak through "symptoms" and be responsive by acknowledging out loud, in our relationships with them, what cannot be spoken: girls' and women's oppression both in their families and by the culture. In reframing their symptoms as a compromise in an effort to resist this oppression – an attempt to connect to a thwarted desire to be a more authentic person – we can aid the young, sagacious and brave girl of earlier years to emerge. I believe that all women carry inside this girl who has been abandoned and betrayed. I suggest that women can receive the support and connection from their female therapists and teachers that can be critical to help them re-engage with the vitality of those earlier years.

REFERENCES

Bernardes, T. (1965). The feminine role: Case report. *Bulletin of The Menninger Clinic, 29*(4), 198-204.

Bernardez, T. (1988). Women and anger: Cultural prohibitions and the feminine ideal. *Work in Progress,* No. 31. Wellesley, MA: Stone Center Working Papers Series.

Brown, L. (1989). *Narratives of relationship: The development of a care voice in girls 7 to 16.* Unpublished doctoral dissertation, Harvard University.

Friedan, B. (1963). *The feminine mystique.* New York: Dell Publishing Co.

Lugones, M. (1990). *Liberatory strategies of the Chicana lesbian: Active subjectivity in the absence of agency.* Paper presented in the Department of Philosophy, Michigan State University.

Gilligan, C., Brown, L. & Rogers, A. (1990). Psyche embedded: A place for body, relationships, and culture in personality theory." In A. Rabin et al. (Eds.), *Studying persons and lives.* New York: Springer.

Paget, M. (1990). Unlearning not to speak. *Human Studies, 13*, 147-161.

Crossing the Desert Alone: An Etiological Model of Female Adolescent Suicidality

James K. Zimmerman

Diane was just about to start her junior year in a demanding, well-respected parochial school in an inner-city neighborhood. She felt confused, faced with the prospect of continuing on a path ostensibly supported by her family – her older twin sisters were both starting their senior year in college – that would simultaneously lead her towards two conflicting outcomes: to an autonomous, independent life and to a widening gulf between her and her mother, who still held to traditional Hispanic cultural values. Additionally, *she* felt little connection to her inner self, to what *she* wanted and what she felt.

One evening, alone in the apartment, Diane swallowed all the pills she could find, including, among others, her father's medication for hypertension. She was found by her parents several hours later and was rushed to a nearby hospital, where she was in intensive care for a week.

* * *

At sixteen years old, Tina thought she had what she wanted: Although she felt little empathic connection with her mother, she had

---

James K. Zimmerman, PhD, is Coordinator of the Adolescent Depression and Suicide Program at Montefiore Medical Center/Albert Einstein College of Medicine. He is also Director of the Brief Treatment/Cognitive Behavioral Specialization in the Child Psychology Internship at Albert Einstein College of Medicine.
His research is supported in part by grants from The Ruane Foundation and the G. Harold and Leila Y. Mathers Charitable Foundation.

found Sara, a woman approximately her mother's age, to whom she could talk intimately and openly. Sara, 33 years old, was pregnant by Juan, who told Tina that he was only with Sara out of a sense of obligation. Soon, Tina and Juan fell in love and began a sexual relationship. Perhaps inevitably, Sara found out. She screamed at Tina, "How could you do this to me!", and then ingested a bottle of ibuprofen before Tina could stop her. Tina called an ambulance, then left to go home when the ambulance arrived. She suddenly realized the impact of her behavior on Sara, and felt deeply guilty. After a call from her mother, who got angry because Tina had been at Sara's apartment in the first place, she took a large quantity of a variety of medications, with the intent to die.

* * *

Sherry was a bright, articulate fourteen-year-old with major behavior problems. At school, she was rebellious and truant; at home, she was emotionally volatile and often stayed out well past midnight. She was sent to live with her father in Florida, but was sent back within a year because she did not get along with her stepmother. Two weeks after she returned to her mother, she was out in front of her apartment at 3 when her stepfather told her to come in. He tried physically to force her inside, at which point she hit him and then ran into the building. An argument over her behavior ensued between her mother, older brother, and stepfather, during which she went into the bathroom and ingested two bottles of pills.

* * *

Suicidality is a serious and pervasive problem among adolescents in American society today. One study, using an anonymous, self-report survey of inner-city teenagers, showed that over sixty percent of the respondents had had suicidal thoughts at some time in their lives, and that nearly nine percent had actually made at least one attempt (Harkavy Friedman, Asnis, Boeck, & DiFiore, 1987). Various researchers and theorists have suggested a number of etiological factors (see Shaffer, 1988, for a review of the literature).

Within the realm of family factors, the following components, among others, have been delineated as contributing to an increased risk of suicidality in adolescents: (1) Symbiotic enmeshment which does not allow for autonomy (Haley, 1980; Pfeffer, 1981, 1986; Spirito, Brown, Overholser, & Fritz, 1989); (2) escalation into crisis at times of life-cycle transitions (Aldridge, 1984; Pfeffer, 1981); (3) intolerance of crisis and crisis management by symptom expression (Aldridge, 1984); and (4) the existence of an "insolvable" problem within the family (Orbach, 1986).

In this paper, I will consider the influence of relational dynamics between mother and daughter, mediated by cultural background, in the etiology of female adolescent suicidality. I will outline the development of suicidality in a particular subgroup of cases seen in a clinic devoted to crisis intervention, brief treatment, and referral for depressed and suicidal teenagers. Specifically, I will focus attention on three adolescent girls who are bright, articulate, and attractive, and who come from Hispanic families in which they represent the hope for the future: the possibility that daughters in the family can succeed where their mothers did not. These girls are targeted by their mothers to become independent, autonomous, and successful (socially and professionally), and to avoid the all-too-prevalent pitfalls of their social environment – early pregnancy, drug and alcohol use, and abusive relationships with men. At the same time, however, they are expected to adhere to more traditional Hispanic female roles, including attributes of obedience, passivity, and valuing highly one's position in the family.

What I will describe below is a theoretical model for the development of suicidality in this subgroup of female adolescents. Central to the model will be the concept of the "insolvable problem" (Orbach, 1986); that is, that these girls feel caught in a dilemma with no apparent solution other than suicide. In addition, I will offer some guidelines for clinical intervention based on this model. The crucial questions I will address are: What brings girls like Diane, Tina, and Sherry, who appear to have more options and opportunities than many others in their environment, to the point of serious attempts to end their lives? What compels them to narrow their options to a single self-destructive act? What are some of the common themes that can help clinicians to prevent recidivism and the possibility that young lives such as these may be prematurely and dramatically ended?

THE MODEL

The model I present includes the following sequence: (1) The presence of "voice" (Gilligan, 1982, 1989) in female adolescents – that is, the unique expression of oneself and one's perspective; (2) the clash of voices of mother and daughter – the struggle between a mother's sense of what her daughter "should" be and what the daughter feels she is; (3) the internalized ambivalence – the girl's internalization of this struggle so that she experiences confusion about who she is and what she should do with her life; (4) the tragic dilemma (or "insolvable" problem (Orbach, 1986)) – the sense that no matter what she does, the adolescent feels she will lose something (either connection with her "voice" or connection with her mother/culture); (5) a perceived moral failure – an event that is construed by the adolescent as representing a failure of either the morality of justice or the morality of care, or both (Gilligan, Brown, and Rogers, 1990); (6) the alliance – an attempt by the daughter to align with the mother's perspective through self-punishment; and (7) the attempted integration – through a suicide attempt, a pathological reconnection with the mother, forcing closer contact and simultaneously promoting apparent autonomy.

The Presence of Voice

Diane, Tina, and Sherry seem to have been in clear contact with their own "voices" – that is, their unique sense of who they are, borne out of their own experience – before adolescence. Both Tina and Sherry were depicted by themselves and their mothers as having been outspoken and strong-willed as younger girls; in fact, they both had had difficulty in school because of this trait. Diane kept in touch with her voice in a more interior way, through journals and withdrawal into a secretive, carefully guarded world in which her inner self could survive (see Gilligan, 1989). According to Gilligan and her colleagues, it is at puberty that some girls begin to experience difficulty in expressing their unique voices in the face of cultural expectations. In fact, the age of thirteen was pinpointed by all three mothers of the girls described here as the beginning of real mother-daughter conflict. By this time, the girls had already begun a desperate struggle to keep in contact with their voices, their sense of self; for Tina and Sherry, this was expressed through acting out, getting in trouble, while Diane attempted to control her experience through further withdrawal.

The Clash of Voices

Gilligan and her colleagues have suggested the use of the language of music in attempting to describe psychological and interpersonal processes (Gilligan, Brown, & Rogers, 1990). In the clash between the girls portrayed here and their mothers, I think a comparison to the music of Charles Ives – characterized by the head-on collision of two distinct, seemingly immutable, mutually excluding, cacophonous voices – best captures the interpersonal dynamics. Just preceding their suicide attempts, both mothers and daughters were blaring out dissonant perspectives on their mutual experience, and neither was able to listen to the other.

In essence, the clash I saw in all three cases was as follows: the girls complained of restrictions by their mothers, of feeling that their mothers were of the "old culture" (i.e., from the island from which they migrated), and that they, the daughters, were American. Diane felt that her mother could not possibly understand her because her mother believed that marriages should be arranged, that boyfriends should ask her permission before dating Diane, and so on. Tina felt her mother was "good at authority but bad at being a friend."

The mothers were also experienced by their daughters as supporting the development of a traditional "care" voice observed in women (Gilligan, 1982), epitomized by interpersonal responsibility, connectedness, and nurturance. However, the emphasis in socializing their daughters appeared to be inclined toward what Gilligan, Brown, and Rogers (1990) refer to as "bad care," in which the girls were expected to focus on the needs of others and the provision of these needs, regardless of the cost to the self. For example, one of the main issues of contention between Tina and her mother was that Tina was expected to care for and be responsible for her eight-year-old sister at all times, but was punished if she disciplined her. For her part, Diane felt compelled to take her mother's needs and demands into account above and before her own.

The Internalized Ambivalence

If all that the mothers of these girls wanted for their daughters was for them to be selfless in their care for others, things would have been simpler. If the mothers had conveyed only the expectation that the girls behave in certain ways dictated by both their native and the American traditional cultural perspectives (i.e, passive, obedient, sexually chaste, "care" oriented), then the essential issue would be the struggle of these adolescent girls against these constraints. Consequently, the girls could have more easily externalized the conflict, adopting an unambivalent, and more typically "adolescent," stance of rebellion against mores experienced as unjust or old-fashioned. Their struggle against acquiescence – the loss of their unique voices – might have been clearer and more self-confident.

In the lives of the three girls I have described here, however, such unidimensionality of maternal expectations was missing. The image projected onto the daughters by their mothers, and ultimately internalized by them, incorporated both the traditional position of female selflessness and the mothers' wish that the daughters would succeed where they did not. These girls were thus encouraged to go to college, fulfill their potential and avoid becoming adolescent mothers: to live out the dream their mothers did not dare believe could come true for themselves.

In essence, then, the mothers' messages are contradictory, and pose for their daughters the nexus of an "insolvable problem" (Orbach, 1986). The mothers' ambivalence about the direction taken in their *own* lives, their *own* struggle between the traditional position and the expression of unique voice, was internalized by their daughters. The central questions – wrestled with internally by the mothers, interpersonally between them and their daughters, and finally internally by the daughters – are these: How can a daughter be passive and compliant and simultaneously fulfill her own unique potential? How can she go beyond her mother and stay in relationship with her at the same time? Paradoxically, to truly succeed in developing and differentiating beyond the boundaries of their families and cultural expectations is to risk losing the connectedness of care and interrelationship. For example, in the midst of her struggle to be able to go out when she wanted to and to begin a career as a performing artist, Diane admitted that she was terrified of losing contact with her family and not knowing where to turn.

The Tragic Dilemma

What invites tragedy in this situation is the dilemma inherent in the struggle between the two apparently contradictory positions of selfless passivity and active, autonomous expression of one's unique voice. Diane was afraid to overtake her mother, to step out into the uncharted territory into which her mother ambivalently thrust her. I imagined the two of them standing at the edge of an endless, searing hot desert, with Diane's mother saying: "Here, I tried to cross it but could not. I had to turn back for lack of water and horses, but I am told there is a world of unimaginable beauty and strength awaiting you on the other side. Now it is your turn to try." Diane gazes out, seeing pearl white bones littering the landscape and vultures waiting sardonically, suspended in the deadly, too-blue sky.

For Diane and the other girls, this choice is too intense, painful, and frightening. This is the point at which the struggle, based on the ambivalence which is in fact within both mother and daughter, ensues in the interpersonal space between them. There are overtones of both the wish for and the fear of true success, and for individuation which is so intense and so common among teenagers on the brink of adulthood. There is the clash, now externalized, between separation and connectedness (Stern, 1989): To feel connected to their mothers at this point means to the girls that they must be what they are told to be, but at the cost of a loss of connectedness to their unique voices, their sense of self. By contrast, metaphorically, to separate is to attempt to cross the desert alone with insufficient water and no navigational aids or orienteering maps; their mothers, constrained by their own experience, cannot provide these supplies, nor do they feel capable of joining their daughters for the trek across. For the girls, to separate is to maintain contact with their pristine, unique voices but to risk losing connectedness with their family and cultural contexts in the process.

Either choice – to cross the desert alone or to remain on the near side of it – risks the loss of connectedness with an aspect of what the daughters have internalized from their mothers. The mothers themselves carry within them the ambivalence experienced by their daughters as well. From this perspective, the daughters' ability to integrate the dilemma would fulfill the mothers' expectations and hopes most fully. However, the complexity of this possibility and the risks involved feel overwhelming to the girls. At this point, the potential for real tragedy – loss inherent in each and every choice – becomes palpably apparent, and, consequently, each girl becomes less clear about who she is and what is right.

In fact, "who she is" becomes the subject of punishment. Diane's mother had begun to refer to her as a "slut" both because she went out to clubs dancing with her older sisters and did not come back until after midnight, and because she had a boyfriend whom she had seen without her mother's permission. Tina's mother told her she was, no good because she would not take care of her younger sister and do the bulk of the housework on a regular basis. Sherry's mother told her she was ruining her (the mother's) life, making her physically ill, by staying out late and "hanging out." The girls interpreted these responses as meaning that they as people were "bad:" unworthy, misunderstood, uncared for. The girls were caught in a dilemma, either "horn" of which was unacceptable and entailed too great a loss. To some extent, they identified with both images their mothers were trying to instill – the passive, obedient, culturally traditional path as well as the independent, successful, culturally superseding one – and could find no way to integrate the two. Again, one "horn" risked loss of self and voice, the other risked loss of cultural connectedness and mother's love; the problem appeared to be truly without solution. Gilligan (1989) summarizes this problem for adolescent girls:

> The central problem - feeling abandoned by others or feeling one should abandon oneself for others - was a problem of disconnection, and often led to desperate actions, desperate efforts at connection. (pp. 8-9)

I suggest that the suicide attempts of Diane, Tina, and Sherry were just such desperate efforts at connection to their mothers, attempts to integrate the contradictory horns of their dilemma.

Perceived Moral Failure

In each case, what ensued in the context of a phase of intense struggle with the dilemma was a triggering event that precipitated the "solution" of a suicide attempt. For Tina, it was the realization that she had betrayed her friend by having a sexual relationship with the father of her friend's baby; for Sherry, it was being the cause of a fight between her brother, mother, and stepfather; and for Diane, it was the idea of returning to a difficult school, which represented the following of her parents' path and the betrayal of her own dream of becoming a performing artist. This type of event as a precipitant of a suicide attempt is not unique to these three cases: A recent actual or perceived social loss or loss of self-esteem has been suggested as one of the common precipitants in attempted and completed suicides in adolescence (Pfeffer, 1986; Shaffer, 1988).

What is essential here is the occurrence of a "perceived moral failure." The term is used in the context of the morality of justice and care described by Gilligan and her colleagues (Brown, 1988; Gilligan, 1989; Gilligan, Brown, & Rogers, 1990). Briefly, care creates and sustains connection and "the care orientation denotes relationships characterized in terms of attachment/detachment" (Brown, 1988, p. 4). The justice orientation is the maintenance of standards of mutual respect and fairness, and "denotes relationships characterized in terms of equality/inequality and reciprocity" (Brown, 1988, p. 4). A moral failure, then, would be an action characterized by either disconnection and abandonment ("bad" care), or by unfairness, lack of respect, or inequality ("bad" justice). The term "perceived" is central because it is the *construing* of an act (not the act itself) by the one who does or experiences it as morally bankrupt, rejecting, or "bad," that precipitates the attempted suicide.

In the cases of the three girls described here, their sense of perceived moral failure stand out in stark relief. Tina's sense of moral failure came from two occurrences in sequence: First, through her realization of her own betrayal of Sara's friendship and trust in having a sexual relationship with Juan, she saw herself as morally bankrupt. She had not felt this relationship was in any way wrong, and, until confronted by Sara, she had justified it by the feeling that she and Juan were in love. After this confrontation, followed by Sara's suicide attempt, Tina felt "hated by everybody." Secondly, when she went home she was unable to reach anyone by telephone which intensified her belief that no one cared about her – that she was abandoned. She then received a call from her mother who was angry at her because she had been with Sara. Tina experienced this as a brutally unempathic, disconnected response to her state of vulnerability, and as a second perceived moral failure; it was within minutes after this call that she ingested "everything she could."

In Sherry's case, the perceived moral failure was experienced in the actions of her stepfather who did not have the right, in her mind, to insist that she come into the apartment, given the fact that her brother had let her stay out late. The sense that her mother was not willing or able to take a stand to protect her against the maltreatment she experienced from her brother multiplied her perception of moral failure in these crucial relationships. On a deeper level, she felt abandoned by her father, who had recently sent her back to live with her mother at the insistence of his new wife. In fact, Sherry's suicide attempt occurred on her father's birthday.

For Tina, then, the perceived moral failures were largely related to disconnection and abandonment (the "care" orientation); for Sherry, there were elements of both the care and justice (fairness, equality) orientations. In Diane's case, the antecedents of her attempt were perhaps more subtle, and certainly less dramatic. She felt disconnection from her mother, who did not support her desire to embark on a performing career, and inequality in that she was not given the level of independence her older sisters had been granted.

In Diane's case, the intensity of the experience of the tragic dilemma, and the relationship between this and the experience of perceived moral failure, was clearest. She was aware not only of needs to hasten her independence and autonomy, but also of being terrified to move on with her life: feeling inadequate to do so and unsupported in her effort. The crux of her perception of her mother's moral failure was that her mother's actions were forcing her to confront her own ambivalence, to struggle with her contradictory internalizations of traditional passivity and unique, autonomous expression of voice.

The intensity of Diane's struggle may explain why she continued to be intermittently suicidal for more than a year, and began several more attempts before actually cutting her wrists fourteen months after her first attempt. This latter attempt followed closely on her parents' announcement that they were considering moving to a Caribbean island within a year; by this time, Diane was quite conscious of being torn between what she saw as irreconcilable simultaneous desires to go to college and get away from her mother and to be passive and to have her mother accessible.

I have focussed attention on Diane at this point because her experience was the most eloquent in expressing the relationship between the tragic dilemma and perceived moral failure. Her perception of moral failure brought her dilemma into stark relief: She could not simultaneously move out on her own, into her own autonomy, and stay connected to traditional passivity and compliance. It was this experience that forced upon her a sense of disconnection, an intensification of the feeling that the problem was unsolvable. Tina experienced this in both the realization of the destructiveness of her relationship with Juan, making her feel that her attempts at autonomy were unacceptable, and in the reaction of her mother, which made her feel that there was no turning back, no connection to be found at home. Sherry's experience closely paralleled Tina's in that her attempt at autonomy – i.e., "hanging out" in front of the building late at night – was not acceptable, nor was her attempt to gain her mother's support and protection.

In each case, the perceived moral failure included the message that the adolescent's voice did not count, or was less important than the needs or demands of her mother and the voice of acculturation. It is this experience that made the girls feel that they could not maintain the level of struggle needed in order to survive. After her second attempt, Diane said, "I don't know who I am, I don't know what to do." She said she had made this attempt because she "couldn't stand the confusion and feeling so bad" about herself.

The Alliance

Immediately preceding the attempted suicides of Tina, Sherry, and Diane, there was a deadly alliance. The ability to withstand the pain of the struggle between maintaining contact with their voices and maintaining connection with their mothers through a traditional passive female stance, suddenly shifted: the girls, in the moment before the attempt, reported feeling that no one cared about them and that they were worthless, lost, and deserving of punishment. The alliance was characterized by a highly confused "desperate effort" to reduce the tension of the impasse between the potential loss of nurturance (from the mother) and the potential loss of nurturance of the self. In the single action of a suicide attempt, there was an effort (1) to "exorcise" and therefore, ironically, to protect the unique voice; and (2) to reject the traditional cultural voice by robbing it of its victim in a pre-emptive meting out of punishment.

Through feeling betrayed or being a betrayer, disconnected from any sense of nurturance or the value of their voices, the girls could not tolerate the continuing tension of their dilemma, their "insolvable" problem. In the moment before the suicide attempt, they had allied with one "horn" of the dilemma: i.e., the perspective embodied in that moment by their mothers' actions and the perception of their mothers' moral failure. From that point of view, the girls' voices were unacceptable and unheard, and therefore worthy of extinction. They wrongly saw their mothers as only supporting the traditional perspective and as unsympathetic to the dilemma that the mothers had also experienced. Confused and alone, the girls tried to reconnect to their mothers by joining them in an act of punishment; the attempt on their own lives was an attempt at reconnection, at solving the dilemma at all costs.

The Attempted Integration

I suggest, then, that the girls' suicide attempts can be understood as desperate efforts to attenuate the clash between their unique voice and the insistent, confining voice of the culture, now felt as personified in their mothers. That is, to end the pain of alienation from their voices and disconnection from their mothers even if it meant dying in the process. Simply put, I see these suicide attempts as problem-solving behaviors. The problem to be solved is the dilemma delineated above; the need is to integrate their unique voice and the wish to connect with their mothers. The desire, then, is to regain the mother's help and support in facing the demands of both American and Hispanic culture and of development into adulthood. In a way, it is a plea for companionship in crossing the desert.

From a more pathological perspective, the suicide attempt also represents a punishment of moral corruption and a "bad" part of the self – either one's unique voice or the now internalized traditional mother. Integration is then to be accomplished by exclusion, by removal of the "bad" part. Tina needed to punish herself for her actions and to punish her mother for not being empathic with her. After her attempt, Tina's mother was angry at her for doing something that so controlled the mother's life and that made her feel like she had to pay attention to Tina all of the time. Tina's suicide attempt thus led to both an intensified connection with her mother and an expression of punitive anger on her mother's part. A similar experience was expressed by Diane's mother. Tina and Diane, for their parts, both felt hounded, intruded upon, harassed by their mothers after the suicide attempt, despite the fact that their mothers gave in to them more afterward. Again, there was an intensified, although unhealthy, connection, as well as a pushing away. The girls felt their mother's concern, expressed in anger, while they could also feel justified in withdrawing – in moving away from their mothers in an apparent shift toward autonomy.

The suicide attempt solves the problem, although in a less than optimal way, by pulling the mother into closer contact through surveillance and worry while simultaneously creating a situation in which the mother, fearful of a repeat attempt, lets her daughter do things more the way she chooses. The irony in this arrangement is that mother and daughter feel connected in a disconnected way – through anger, intrusion, and perceived exploitation. Both experience this circumstance as unfair. The daughter feels harassed and the mother feels she must "walk on eggshells," as Tina's mother described it.

THE DESERT REVISITED

In briefly delineating the above etiological model of a pathway to suicide in Hispanic female adolescents, I raise as many questions as I answer. Clearly, Diane, Tina, and Sherry found themselves in the midst of such intense struggles in part because they were able to envision a life for themselves "beyond the desert," and because they were exquisitely sensitive to the dilemma which fueled the struggle itself. It is an open question whether or not such dynamics apply to girls of other cultural backgrounds, to adolescent females in general (but with differing levels of intensity and response), or to adolescent males at all.

Perhaps a more crucial question is whether the desert must be crossed alone, or if ways of relating between mother and daughter can create a mutual, shared crossing, such that the girl can maintain contact with her unique voice and with the voice(s) of the culture without losing connection with either vital source of nurturance.

TREATMENT

Whether the desert must be crossed alone or can be crossed in relationship with another, it is clear that a way of assisting adolescent girls in managing this experience is to help them titrate the experience of the dilemma so that the ambivalence – the terrifying potential for loss in one or the other direction – can be identified and tolerated. Adaptive strategies can be developed that will function like proper desert-crossing supplies and equipment. What, then, can be done in psychotherapy to defuse the kind of situation described above so that both mother and daughter regain a sense of empathic connection and reciprocity? I will present three techniques briefly here: (1) Delineating the dilemma; (2) Promoting authorship of and listening to narrative (Tappan & Brown, 1989); and (3) Reorienting to "good care" and "good justice" (Gilligan, Brown, & Rogers, 1990).

Delineating the Dilemma

An essential early phase of treatment includes helping both mother and daughter identify and clarify the dilemma in their own terms. In this regard, I bring mother and daughter into a session together. A major thrust of this intervention is to "depathologize" the suicide attempt and remove the interplay of blame and guilt that so often follows from it. For example, it was vital for Diane to be able to describe to her mother the pain of trying to establish and maintain her sense of self in the face of an intense need to feel her mother's presence and potential for nurturance. It was also important for her to be able to tell her mother that her more "American" ways of behaving were not intended to be hurtful or rejecting, but were necessary for her ability to evolve in her own uniqueness. Delineating the dilemma allowed her to speak of her need for a separateness that was not experienced as hurtful, so that she could "survive and at the same time not damage her mother and incur retributive anger and rejection."

Tina and her mother were intensely engaged in a "dance" of intrusion, exploitation and mistrust. Early in treatment, Tina made it clear that she needed her mother to show her "softness" and vulnerability, but not to "breathe down her neck" with angry worry. She needed her mother to trust her to manage her own life, but to understand simultaneously how important it was that they be able to speak and listen openly to one another. Tina used the word "sisters" to describe the experience for which she longed: she wished that they could communicate with care, thus maintaining connection, but with the concomitant individuation that is needed for two individuals to be in a mature relationship with each other.

Promoting Authorship of Narrative

Tappan and Brown state: "Individuals develop morally by 'authoring' their own moral stories" (Tappan & Brown, 1989, p. 183), and that "a narrative might well be considered a solution to . . . the problem of how to translate knowing into telling" (p. 185). One of the consistently restorative, integrating experiences I used in the psychotherapy of the girls and their mothers was to have each of them tell their experience of the suicide attempt and events surrounding it – with the other asked to "just listen carefully." Each is then able to "translate knowing into telling," both for herself and for the other, and each is also able to gain empathic entry to the other's experience of the events. What follows is often a deeply emotional experience of reconnection between mother and daughter.

In Tina's case, her mother's description of seeing her in the hospital brought tears to Tina's eyes, both in recognition of the pain her mother had gone through, and in experiencing the connectedness her mother actually felt with her. This moment in treatment was a turning point, after which Tina was clear that she would not resort to suicidal behavior as a form of communication or problem-solving. It also allowed her mother to trust her to a greater extent, which relieved the burden of stress for both of them.

Not only is the relationship between mother and daughter strengthened, but it is also the case that the telling and listening to the narrative helps each to feel more integrated as a unique self, more in touch with her "voice." "Authorship not only expresses itself through narrative, it also develops through narrative" (Tappan & Brown, 1989, p. 192); and "to narrate a story is already to reflect upon the event narrated" (Ricoeur, 1986, p. 61, cited in Tappan & Brown, 1989). Through telling, then, an individual owns experience, understands it, comes to terms with it. The process of narrating becomes a crucial restorative, reintegrative function for both mother and daughter after a girl's suicide attempt.

Reorienting to "Good" Care and "Good" Justice

Through delineating the dilemma and authoring the narrative, the girls and their mothers were enabled to rediscover a more positive connectedness and sense of reciprocity. Through this reconnection to each other, feelings of intrusion and exploitation were replaced by understanding and empathy; feelings of inequality and unfairness were transmuted into a sense of mutual respect. For example, a turning point in treatment for Sherry was the realization by her mother that Sherry needed her mother's protection from the chaotic environment in which they lived. When Sherry's mother told the other, more transient members of the household that this was *her* house and Sherry's house – taking a stand which definitively conveyed a concern for her daughter's welfare – Sherry's school attendance and work improved, and she stopped "hanging out on the stoop" as much. Furthermore, she was able to be more supportive of her mother's struggle to keep career and home life together. For Diane, it was the realization of the contribution of her own withdrawn, moody behavior to her mother's overbearingness that made her able to communicate more directly, which in turn allowed her mother to trust her and "back off" to some extent.

CONCLUSION

The basic therapeutic intent of the techniques I briefly described above is to help both mother and daughter to integrate the experience of the daughter's suicide attempt and to understand it in the context of a developmental and moral dilemma. What is hoped is that identifying the dilemma and narrating and listening to each other's experiences in treatment will lead to a greater degree of both connectedness and separateness, of empathic understanding which fosters the ability to be openly nurturant while providing enough distance to experience companionship without enmeshment. This psychotherapeutic intervention is a strategy by which daughter and mother can make the attempt to cross the desert together. Thus the adolescent can feel supported by her mother in the journey toward a both caring and autonomous adulthood and deepened self-understanding.

REFERENCES

Aldridge, D. (1984). Family interactions and suicidal behavior: A brief review. *Journal of Family Therapy, 6,* 309-322.

Brown, L. (Ed.) (1988). *A guide to reading narratives of conflict and choice for self and moral voice.* (Monograph No. 1). Cambridge, MA: The Center for the Study of Gender, Education and Human Development, Harvard University.

Gilligan, C. (1982). *In a different voice: Psychological theory and women's development.* Cambridge, MA: Harvard University Press.

Gilligan, C. (1989). Teaching Shakespeare's sister. In C. Gilligan, N. Lyons, & T.

Hanmer (Eds.), *Making connections: The relational worlds of adolescent girls at Emma Willard School.* Troy, NY: Emma Willard School.

Gilligan, C., Brown, L. M., & Rogers, A. G. (1990). Psyche embedded: A place for body, relationships, and culture in personality theory. In A. Rabin et al. (Eds.), *Studying persons and lives.* New York: Springer.

Haley, J. (1980). *Leaving Home.* New York: McGraw-Hill.

Harkavy Friedman, J. M., Asnis, G. M., Boeck, M., & DiFiore, J. (1987). The prevalence of specific suicidal behaviors: A high school sample. *American Journal of Psychiatry, 144,* 1203-1206.

Orbach, I. (1986). The 'insolvable problem' as a determinant in the dynamics of suicidal behavior in children. *Journal of American Psychotherapy, 40*(4), 511-520.

Pfeffer, C. R. (1981). The family system of suicidal children. *American Journal of Psychotherapy, 35*(3), 330-341.

Pfeffer, C. R. (1986). *The suicidal child.* New York: Guilford Press.

Ricoeur, P. (1986). *Time and narrative: Volume 2.* Chicago: University of Chicago Press.

Shaffer, D. (1988). The epidemiology of teen suicide: An examination of risk factors. *Journal of Clinical Psychiatry, 49*(9), 36-41.

Spirito, A., Brown, L., Overholser, J., & Fritz, G. (1989). Attempted suicide in adolescence: A review and critique of the literature. *Clinical Psychology Review, 9,* 335-363.

Stern, L. (1989). Conceptions of separation and connection in female adolescents. In C. Gilligan, N. Lyons, & T. Hanmer (Eds.), *Making connections: The relational worlds of adolescent girls at Emma Wihard School.* Troy, NY: Emma Willard School.

Tappan, M., & Brown, L. (1989). Stories told and lessons learned: Toward a narrative approach to moral development and moral education. *Harvard Educational Review, 59*(2), 182-205.

Working with Adolescent Girls: Strategies to Address Health Status

Christine Renee Robinson

> What is unvoiced or unspoken, because it is out of relationship, tends to get out of perspective and to dominate psychic life. (Gilligan, 1990a, p. 511)

There is distressing truth to this statement, a concern that resonates for all who work with or know adolescent girls. By not speaking to girls about health and their changing bodies, women and men are sending a powerful lifelong message that travels generation to generation, about our culture, our values, our lives, and our fears. Though we live in our bodies for our entire lives, the connection between the emotional and physical realm remains a mystery for most of us. Through our lack of information, our discomfort and silence, we are teaching adolescent girls to deny, misunderstand, and ignore a fundamental part of their lives: their bodies.

As a professional researcher in developmental psychology and as a public health analyst administering programs that serve hundreds of girls across the state of Massachusetts, I am greatly disturbed by the findings of Gilligan and her colleagues at the Project on the Psychology of Women and the Development of Girls at Harvard University. The loss of "voice," the loss of "truth," and what seems to be an acquiescence to "norms" of Western Culture has been observed by these researchers as girls move from girlhood to adolescence (Brown 1989, in press; Gilligan, 1990a, 1990b; Rogers, 1990; Rogers & Gilligan, 1988). Developmentally, early adolescence is a time of newness, a time of multiple, novel, stressful

---

Christine Renee Robinson is Director of the Division for School Age and Adolescent Health, Department of Public Health, Commonwealth of Massachusetts.

challenges. Girls who enter the early adolescent period with misinformation, or no information about their bodies, development, and health needs, find the negotiation of this critical period problematic. Other researchers have noted that serious problems such as school dropout, substance abuse, pregnancy, and suicide have their initiation and show up in rising rates among younger teens (Hamburg, 1990). Perhaps reflecting but also contributing to these problems, teens are stereotyped as wild, focused on sexuality, pleasure seeking, with no positive role in our society (Nightengale & Wolverton, 1988).

The World Health Organization defines "health" as a state of complete physical, mental and social well-being. Using this definition as a criterion for health, a "healthy" transition from childhood to adulthood in today's society is difficult. Developmental psychology tells us that adolescents are in a period of dynamic physical and psychosocial maturation. Physical changes in growth and sexual maturity are accompanied by changes in self-concept (Petersen, 1988); psychological changes include both cognitive maturation from concrete to abstract thinking and the mastering of specific developmental tasks (Kagan, 1972). Challenges of achievement in school are accompanied by increases in autonomy and expectations of independence. Personal and social values become more differentiated as decisions about health, substance use, sex roles and achievement all are shaped during this critical period (Hamburg & Takanishi, 1989). At the same time, sexual development and sexuality are accompanied by changes in intimate relationships and personal commitment. Lack of information and misinformation, the physical and/or psychological experience of poverty and racism can significantly hinder the accomplishment of these essential tasks. Developing a moral character and a functional personal value system is also difficult, especially with the pervasive influence of print and visual media.

As I look at statewide trends in Massachusetts and national trends, the current state of adolescent health is troubling. As health care administrators, parents, teachers, and mental health professionals, it is imperative that we be more honest with girls to prepare them to face reality. As a culture we tend to protect our children, especially girls, as opposed to *preparing* them. The realities of violence, poverty, and substance abuse are ugly, yet they have become part of the daily reality of many of our girls' lives. Our communication and language must welcome questions, provide the answers we have, and convey a willingness to learn with young women. To this end, comprehensive health education in schools grades K-12 needs to be revolutionized to be inclusive, multicultural, and to address issues such as violence, substance abuse, racism, and also to offer instructive work in responsible decision making techniques. As these programs are developed to be empathetic with adolescents' experiences and to strengthen social support for adolescents, they also will be able to encourage positive roles for adolescents in our culture. For all of these reasons, access to comprehensive health care services should be provided for teens, and school-based health centers provide a sound model. To assist adolescent girls in finding roles in society that are self expressive and that are appreciated, we need to find ways to assist girls in resisting debilitating and dangerous conventions of femininity, and to resist ignorance about their own bodies which serves to harm them. It is critical to empower them with honest relationships and trustworthy information.

THE NEED FOR CONCERN: ADOLESCENT HEALTH STATUS AND ACCESS TO HEALTH CARE

There is a crisis among adolescents, a health crisis. Daily in my work I note that life is grim for large numbers of teens, male and female, urban, suburban, and rural; teens of all races, languages and ancestry. Adolescents are the only age group in this country whose mortality rate has *increased* over the last thirty years. Increases in adolescent mortality rates have been accompanied by a shift in the causes of mortality rates from those due to disease to those related to social, environmental and behavioral factors (Millstein, 1988). Shifts in the causes of mortality in youth have been accompanied by changes in the causes of morbidity as well. The new morbidities of adolescents include injury associated with the use of motor and recreational vehicles, substance use, and consequences of sexual activity such as pregnancy and sexually transmitted diseases (Centers for Disease Control, 1982; Johnston et al.,

1984; Shafer & Irwin, 1983). The 1978 President's Commission on Mental Health Task Force on Infants, Children and Adolescents viewed adolescents as one of the most underserved groups in the United States. In 1986, the Office of Technology Assessment estimated that at least 12% of the nation's children were in need of some type of mental health treatment, but fewer than one third of those who needed it received any treatment. Mental health services for adolescents often have long waiting lists.

Adolescent health and medicine have come to the forefront recently. The "newness" of this area is evident in the various ways statistics regarding adolescent health are tabulated. Many data sources merge children and adolescents, creating an aggregate total of those aged 1 to 18. More sources are beginning to differentiate certain conditions by age. Age specific data is available for the more prevalent causes of morbidity such as pregnancy and vehicular accidents. Still, the existing data are useful to illustrate health trends among adolescents. These trends are generalizable and yield significant information related to the lives of girls and young women. I have selected a few national and statewide statistics which highlight the precarious condition of adolescents.

National Data:

- Every eight seconds of the school day, an American child drops out of school.
- Every seven minutes, an American child is arrested for a drug offense.
- Every 53 minutes, an American child dies because of poverty.
- Every 36 minutes, an American child is killed or injured by guns.
- Every 78 seconds an adolescent attempts suicide.
- Every 90 minutes one attempted adolescent suicide is successful.
- Every 20 minutes an adolescent is killed in an automobile accident.
- Every 80 minutes an adolescent is a victim of homicide.
- Every 31 seconds an adolescent gets pregnant.
- Every 26 seconds of each day, an American child runs away from home.

(Children's Defense Fund, 1990.)

- Out of the average high school graduating class of 40, 36 have used alcohol, 8 have used cocaine, 11 have smoked marijuana, 1 has used heroin, 15 live in poverty, 6 have run away, 4 dropped out before graduation, 2 gave birth before graduation, 1 attempted suicide. (Novello, 1989).
- Sexually transmitted disease rates are higher among adolescents than any other age group; one-fourth of adolescents are infected with a sexually transmitted disease before graduating from high school. (National Institutes on Allergies and Infectious Disease Study Group, 1980.)
- By 1989, the United States had become home to more than 100,000 street gangs with a combined membership of nearly 1.5 million youths and adults (Delattre, 1990).
- Adolescents between the ages of 11 and 20 visited physicians' offices less often then any other group although they have a higher rate of acute conditions such as infections, influenza, and injuries (Cypress, 1984).

Statewide Trends:

- On average, one in seven adolescents in Massachusetts has had one sexually transmitted disease in the past year (Massachusetts Department of Public Health, 1990).
- Half of all survivors of sexual assault in Massachusetts were under 18 years of age at the time of the latest sexual assault (MDPH, 1990).

Study of physiology and psychology tell us that puberty is not only life changing but also is unpredictable in timing of onset or in rates of physical change. Adolescent girls may perceive that their bodily changes are too early, too late, or abnormal (Blyth, Simmons, & Zakin, 1985; Brooks-Gunn & Warren, 1988; Greif & Ulman, 1982; Rierdan & Koff, 1980). Yet trends are consistent: concerns over body image are pervasive (Freedman, 1984). Young adolescents have deep concerns about their physical attractiveness and often feel vulnerable to the accompanying changes of temperament. At the same time, young adolescents have relatively little information about the wide range of normalcy or the varying timetables or patterns of physical changes. Thus adolescent girls are physically mature, without understanding the significance of their development. The prevalence of provocative sexual imagery, often directed at teenagers by TV and movie programs, tends to exacerbate the situation. Early adolescents are both ignorant and have misinformation about sexuality, sexually transmitted diseases and AIDS. They are unprepared for peer pressures regarding sex. They need to understand puberty, to learn about human biology and to be educated about important health issues and health related behaviors (Hamburg, 1990).

According to a World Health Organization classification, teens suffer from four types of health problems: those related to growth and development, risk taking behavior and violence, sexuality, and the psychological transition to adulthood. Working with adolescent girls I observe a daily struggle with developmental issues. They are acquiring the ability to ask for help and the skills to know when help is needed. And yet in many ways these girls are learning that to ask for help is childish and not adult behavior. This developmental dilemma compounded by silence, rampant misinformation, and self-diagnosis leaves girls in an extremely precarious position, especially in early adolescence.

At present many adolescent girls face barriers to health care and to information. The cost of health care is high, and increasing numbers of Americans are unable to afford it. The number of children living in poverty continues to increase dramatically, and many are not eligible for Medicaid because of restrictive eligibility requirement. Many insurance programs cover care only in the event of illness of hospitalization, leaving families responsible for routine physicals and well child care as well as a portion of other medical expenses. Physician's hours and clinics are open primarily during school hours, and transportation is often a problem for both urban and rural teens.

We live in a culture which denies the reality of poverty, sexism, racism, and sexual abuse; a culture which glorifies violence, and has no voice, language or process to prepare adolescents, particularly adolescent girls, for the future. There is a discomfort in naming body parts and functions, and a greater discomfort in teaching adolescent girls their right to resist the subtle oppression of acquiescence.

How do we develop a more relational language, one that has comfort in expressing our physical and emotional realities? If we want girls to grow into women who have reciprocal, respectful, non-violent, loving relationships, how can we give them the tools to build those relationships, and recognize the pitfalls?

DEVELOPING A RESPONSE TO A CRISIS IN HEALTH CARE

In general, American families communicate about sexuality infrequently, and these occasional conversations are all too often awkward and incomplete. When children are young, parents are reluctant to raise many issues related to love, intimacy, or eroticism. Parents wait for children to ask, and while they are waiting, children are learning not to ask questions because no one talks about "those things." During adolescence girls are more likely than boys to be recipients of control messages: 'shoulds' and 'should nots' are frequent, and information is often delivered to girls with a bias (Kahn & Smith, 1989). Specifically, in the Western Culture there is great discomfort in discussing the body, our physical reality, and in discussing our emotions and how we respond to them. Topics such as contraception, nudity, and masturbation continue to be taboo (Kahn & Smith, 1989), while emotional issues such as love, intimacy, and what happens on a date are rarely mentioned.

While families are changing, becoming less multigenerational, more mobile, and smaller, other social and community institutions vital to the successful development of adolescents are also experiencing major challenges. New demands are being placed on schools to strengthen their core educational mission, while at the same time they are expected to fulfill a variety of other needs. These critical social institutions, the school and the family, need strengthening if they are to provide the support that adolescents so badly need as they negotiate the transition to adulthood.

The response to health problems has usually not been multidisciplinary nor consistent. Most frequently in this culture, we have tried to isolate a problem, deny its existence, and then "prevent it" or more accurately, respond to it. This has been the pattern in "preventing" running away, "preventing" teenage pregnancy, and "preventing" alcohol abuse. The statistics presented earlier give some indication that this method is not successful. In this so-called prevention mind set, we have lost sight of our own participation in and perpetuation of the current problems. We have also lost sight of the fact that we should be preparing a future generation who will be responsible for raising the next generation. By not talking and not teaching, we *are* teaching denial. Adolescent girls hear our silence and sense our discomfort; in addition they are learning from us how adults respond to teenage girls. How can we then encourage health among teenage girls?

School-based health centers offer a model of health care that is multidisciplinary, addresses many needs simultaneously, and also draws on existing community networks. School-based health centers in Massachusetts for example strive to promote a multidisciplinary collaborative team approach to the provision of health care. They provide social supports as well as health care, thereby increasing the probability that students will remain in school. Extensive networking with a wide array of existing community resources to mobilize and maximize available services for teens is an ongoing process inherent in the work of these centers. The role of the school-based health center is to facilitate networking between students, schools, parents, and the community.

School-based health centers also constitute a supportive link between the school and the health care system. As Millstein (1988) notes,

> The school system and its personnel play a crucial role in the acceptance of school-linked centers by students, parents and the community. Health education has traditionally been the responsibility of the schools, who may or may not have the resources to provide well-developed, appropriate curriculum in this area. With the presence of school-linked health centers, schools have the potential to strengthen their health education programs. . . . (p. 23)

In Massachusetts centers, education and counseling are provided at the same time as medical services. Zabin et al. (1986) found that young people will rarely return to a site for education if they have already received the medical services they need. Second, "teenagers appear to need the support of the same professional over time. The consistency of a relationship builds trust, thus allowing the adolescent to synthesize what he/she had learned and return to share private concerns" (p. 78). School based health centers provide continuity of care and consistency of providers. All school based health centers in Massachusetts are linked with a community hospital, health center, or board of health which provides year round access and continuity with the same provider. For adolescents, and particularly adolescent girls, the relationship formed with a health care provider is a source of much needed information. Mobilizing broad based community support for school-based centers is also crucial. Community groups need to be involved from the initial stages and their concerns addressed. Specific individuals and groups who play a special role in assuring successful implementation include parents, school personnel, school administrators, youth-serving agencies, clergy, the business community and health care providers. Organizing a community wide advisory board is a common method of assuring continuing community input and support for the health center. In addition to offering support and guidance and helping to identify funding sources, advisory groups can play an important role in public relations. There is an ongoing need to heighten public awareness of the health care needs of adolescents. Public interest arid support are essential as we address the health care needs of girls.

CONCLUSION

As the adults who work with girls, who parent girls, and as women who were once girls, we must cease to protect our girls and *prepare* them. We must give them frank information, foster responsible risk taking and provide opportunities for mastery, to prepare them to face reality. Today's realities of violence, poverty, and substance abuse do not have to be the reality of tomorrow. To the degree that they may be, we will have given girls tools to recognize and address them. By providing comprehensive health education that is inclusive and culturally sensitive in grades K-12, and teaching responsible decision making techniques, we are beginning to broaden our own communication and willingness to learn with our young women. School based health centers provide a sound model of accessible health care and an empathetic supportive forum for leadership.

If we can prepare young women in these ways, we begin to foster an environment where girls can resist unhealthy conventions of femininity. We begin to support adolescent girls as they continue to question, and continue to explore the reality of the world as they see it. It may be true that as adults we have more of an understanding of the process of puberty and their rapidly changing lives, but our willingness to share this knowledge honestly and totally and to build a bridge of preparation is essential. As adults it is critical that we give adolescent girls the information which is so crucial to their future and answers to their very real questions and concerns.

REFERENCES

Blyth, D., Simmons, R., & Zakin, D. (1985). Satisfaction with body image for early adolescent females: The impact of pubertal timing within different school environments. *Journal of Youth and Adolescence. 14*(3), 207-225.

Brooks-Gunn, J., & Warren, M. (1988). The psychological significance of secondary sexual characteristics in nine- to eleven-year-old girls. *Child Development, 59*, 1061-1069.

Brown, L. (1989) *Narratives of relationship: The development of a care voice in girls ages 7 to 16.* Unpublished doctoral dissertation, Harvard University.

Brown, L. (in press). A problem of vision: the development of relational voice in girls ages 7 to 16. *Women's Studies Quarterly.*

Children's Defense Fund. (1990). S.O.S. *America: A children's defense budget.* Washington, DC: Author.

Centers for Disease Control. (1982). Accidental injury in the U.S. *Morbidiry and Mortality Weekly Review,* 31:110-1.

Cypress, B.K. (1984, September). Health care of adolescents by office-based physicians: National Ambulatory Care Survey, 1980-81. (Publication No. 99). United States Department of Health and Human Services, Advance data, NCHS.

Delattre, E. (1990, November). *Ethics and urban gang tyranny: Betrayal of our children.* Olin Public Lecture Series, Boston University, School of Education, Boston, MA.

Freedman, R. (1984). Reflections on beauty as it related to health in adolescent females. In S. Golub (Ed.), *Health care of the female adolescent.* (pp. xx) New York, NY: The Haworth Press, Inc.

Gilligan, C. (1990a). Joining the resistance: Psychology, politics, girls and women. *Michigan Quarterly Review, 29*(4), 501-536.

Gilligan, C. (1990b). Teaching Shakespeare's sister: Notes from the underground of female adolescence. In C. Gilligan, N. Lyons, & T. Hanmer (Eds.), *Making connections: The relational worlds of adolescent girls at Emma Willard School* (pp. 6-29). Cambridge, MA: Harvard University Press.

Greif, E., & Ulman, K. (1982). The psychological impact of menarche on early adolescent females: A review of the literature. *Child Development, 53,* 1413-1430.

Hamburg, B.A. (1974). Early adolescence: A specific and stressful stage of the life cycle. In G.V. Coelno, D.A. Hamburg & J.E. Adams (Eds), *Coping and adaptation.* (pp. xx) New York: Basic Books.

Hamburg, B.A. (1990). Life skills training: Preventive interventions for young adolescents. Carnegie Council on Adolescent Development, Carnegie Corporation, NY.

Hamburg, B.A., & Takanishi, R. (1989). Preparing for life. *American Psychologist,* May, 825-827. (Vol. 44 No. 5)

Johnston, L.D., Bachman, J.G., & O'Malley, P.M. (1984). *Use of licit and illicit drugs by America's high school students, 1975-84* (Publication No. 85-1394). Rockville, MD: United States Department of Health and Human Services, National Institute of Drug Abuse.

Kagan, J. (1972). A conception of early adolescence. In J. Kagan & R. Coles (Eds.), *12 to 16: Early adolescence* (pp. 90-105). New York: Norton.

Kahn, J., & Smith, K. (1989). *Familial Communication and Adolescent Sexual Behavior*, American Institutes for Research, Cambridge, MA, 1984.

Massachusetts Department of Public Health. (1990, February). *Shattering the Myths: Sexual Assault in Massachusetts 1985-1987.* Boston: Author.

Massachusetts Department of Public Health. (1990). *Teens at Risk: STD and AIDS.* Boston: Author.

Millstein, S.G. (1988). The potential of school-linked centers to promote adolescent health and development. Washington, DC: Carnegie Council on Adolescent Development.

National Institutes on Allergies and Infectious Disease Study Group. (1980). *Sexually Transmitted Diseases – Summary and Recommendations.* Washington, DC: United States Department of Health, Education, and Welfare, National Institutes of Health.

Nightengale, E.O., & Wolverton, L. (1988). Adolescent rolelessness in modern society. Invited address for the American Medical Association, *National Congress on Adolescent Health: Charting a course through turbulent times.* Chicago, IL.

Novello, A. (1989, March). Recommendations to states from the chairman of the Secretary's Health and Human Services work group on pediatric HIV infection and disease. Presented at: Pediatric AIDS: Planning a Family Centered Action Continuum, Nashua, NH.

Office of Technology Assessment. (1986). *Children's Mental Health: Problems and Services.* Washington, DC: U.S. Government Printing Office.

Petersen, A.C. (1988). Adolescent development. *Annual Review of Psychology, 39*, 583-607.

President's Commission on Mental Health. (1978). *Report to the President from the President's Commission on Mental Health.* Washington, DC: U.S. Government Printing Office.

Rierdan, J., & Koff, E. (1980). Representation of the female body by early and late adolescent girls. *Journal of Youth and Adolescence. 9*(4), 339-346.

Rogers, A. (1990). The development of courage in girls and women. Unpublished manuscript, Harvard University, Project on the Psychology of Women and the Development of Girls, Cambridge, MA.

Rogers, A., & Gilligan, C. (1988). *Translating the language of adolescent girls: Themes of moral voice and stages of ego development* (Monograph No. 6). Cambridge, MA: Project on the Psychology of Women and the Development of Girls, Harvard Graduate School of Education.

Shafer, M.A., & Irwin, C.E. (1983). Sexually transmitted diseases in adolescents. In M. Green & R.J. Haggerty (Eds.), *Ambulatory pediatrics, III.* (pp. xx) Philadelphia: W.B. Saunders Press.

Zabin, L., Hirsch, M., Smith, E., Street, R., & Hardy, J. (1986). Adolescent pregnancy-prevention program: A model for research and evaluation. *Journal of Adolescent Health Care, 7*, 77-87.

When the Body Speaks: Girls, Eating Disorders and Psychotherapy

Catherine Steiner-Adair

In teenage girls' struggle with their bodies and eating disorders, I see a joining of the psychological and political drama in a struggle around resistance (Gilligan, 1989). Girls and women, and the culture at large in which they are embedded, hate what is symbolically associated with the rounded woman's body, the fundamental importance of (inter) dependence (symbolized in the pregnant body) and the necessary experience of self in connection (Miller, 1984; Surrey, 1985) found only in relationships (Steiner-Adair, 1986). Research on the values and personality traits associated with thin female bodies present the patriarchal values that dominate psychological theory as well as the white male power base: independence, self assertion, aggressiveness, autonomy, mind over matter, absence of dependency and need (Boskind-Lodahl, 1976; Steiner-Adair, 1989; Wooley, Wooley & Dyrenforth, 1979). When I look at eating disorders as a body politic, rather than a body pathological, eating disorders become a symbol of a culture that does not support female development and symbolically outcasts that which is central to female identity and mature adulthood (Steiner-Adair, 1986). Ariel, a sixteen year old girl whom I have known for two and a half years, writes in her journal:

Catherine Steiner-Adair, EdD, is a practicing licensed psychologist. She is a member of the Harvard Project on the Psychology of Women and the Development of Girls, and adjunct teaching faculty at The Family Institute of Cambridge. She has written a series of articles on the psychology of women, psychotherapy, and eating disorders.

> My body tenses as I hurl the textured glass into the ancient porcelain sink. Random chunks splatter throughout the dark steamy room as I thunk down to the floor. Yellow bile coats the slimy, ridged roof of my mouth. The consistency of it and the retched taste cause me to vomit uncontrollably onto the cool seaweed green tile floor. Angry, dizzy, hopeless tears make puddles in the now orangey mass of sticky liquids. I stare hatefully at my crumpled body still gasping for air and cry repulsed and enraged. I feel trapped. I can no longer run from the pain that keeps biting me with its sharpened fangs. I'm so tired, there is so little left of me. I'm no longer anything but a facade only trying to meet unreal expectations. Expectations that try to force me into a mold I can't fit into. Why can't I just be me?
>
> Why do you constantly contradict everything that I believe? Am I always wrong? I respect you so little, yet your opinions mean so much to me. I feel so abused and simultaneously so greedy. How can I want more? Why do I need so much? Why am I never enough? Why am I not good enough to deserve what I so desperately need from you?
>
> I need to be listened to, not neglected. I need to be dealt with as a caring, real person, not just a stereotype. I need affection from both of you. I need you to acknowledge that I am right when I am. You should both be able to admit that you are wrong sometimes. You are not perfect. Don't always react to me with fragile self confidence. Don't make me rebel against you. Free me, trust me and care about me at the same time. Yes, I know that this is too much to ask. I always want too much of everything. I'm sorry. I don't mean to make you feel inadequate.
>
> I feel so weak, so tired, so faded, so abandoned. Why did I want to grow up? I'm so alone.

When Ariel first came to therapy, she was vomiting twice a day, very depressed and disgusted with herself, and violently trying to fit her body into a mold to which it could not conform. I asked Ariel to write about her binge. I did not ask her not to binge, because I wanted her to discover the meaning of her behavior, to understand what she was trying to say with her body. She had long ago lost the ability to speak directly with her words, for as she writes, her answers and her beliefs, her feelings, are never listened to or respected.

For girls like Ariel who struggle with eating disorders, their bodies become the self that speaks. What Ariel can not say directly or consciously, she speaks symbolically. I try to convey my respect by not ignoring the symptom by trying to get rid of it (with cognitive behavioral techniques). Ariel and I have listened to her self speaking through her body and understand her attempt to communicate through her behavior. I tell her that I believe there is integrity in her attempt to speak through her illness, but because she has been so silenced and isolated, her message has been lost to her in self-destructive behavior.

If I listen to Ariel's words, I hear her body speaking a resistance that she fears saying directly "I can't fit." She tells me that her eating disorder is the punishment she deals herself for resisting, for not wanting to fit. It is the pain that keeps "biting" her. Ariel begins therapy in a state of physical exhaustion. Along with her binging and vomiting, she exercises with a vengeance. In the early meetings, she also talks about running away, killing herself. At this juncture in therapy, she feels angry, dizzy, hopeless. I hear in the progression of her adjectives, a familiar path away from clarity, away from knowing what she knows. Like other teenage girls with eating disorders, she truly hates herself as well as her body. She knows that she hates being a girl as well: "I hate being a girl, I wish I was a boy. It sucks being a girl. You get totally put down, sexually harassed, ditzed." Ariel's rage and repulsion are not only directed outward to those who create the molds, those who contradict, disqualify and refuse to listen to her but she also tortures herself with self denigrating words and self destructive behavior. These are attempts to solve what feels to Ariel like a hopelessly impossible situation. She asks herself, "How can I grow up and be myself without fitting myself into molds that do not fit me?'

In therapy, I ask Ariel to put words and feelings to her actions. I tell her that she is trying to say some essential truths about herself that she has lost the ability to say directly. I ask her to begin with becoming aware of her body. When she writes about binging and vomiting, this is her first report from the "front," the first report from a rebel in the bathroom. Ariel understands that the scene is her body and it is her mouth that would speak if it could directly. She knows that the audience is herself and me. However, as soon as she comes up against her anger, it dissipates into dizziness, tears, and finally hopelessness: Her outwardly directed resistance disappears, and instead she hates herself.

The illness catches her and silences her. An excellent example of what war psychologists call internal desertion. Ariel, like the soldier who loses sight of who the enemy is and thinks it is him or herself, begins to criticize herself – "I know I ask too much" "I don't deserve . . . " "I am not enough . . . " "I am not good enough to deserve simple basic needs." She undermines herself and turns on her own needs. She struggles to talk directly to "you," but she sinks into a one down position. She sounds to herself like a petulant unreasonable little girl.

SPEAKING IN THERAPY

I believe that part of the reason Ariel is so caught up in her eating disorder is that she has come to believe that the only way she can approach asking for what she needs is to ask from this position of illness. When I think about the enormous physical and psychic pain Ariel lives with, I find myself playing with the etymological roots of her contemporary diagnosis. Eating means two things, I recall: to take in by mouth – and to destroy. Why is Ariel living in the double meanings simultaneously with binging and vomiting. What is the order, the social patterns and hierarchy that she must dispel, do the opposite of? I think this is about the molds, the unresolvable conflict she experiences between growing up and fitting into the expectations, the molds, continuing to be herself, and continuing to live fully in her body as she struggles in the world as an adolescent girl.

Key questions in therapy become, can I say what I think and feel as a woman in the world and still be safe and respected? Do I have to remove bodily parts of myself that are stereotypically feminine in order to be successful in work and attaining relationships? If I am to empower myself, must I betray myself also, my vulnerability, my need to nurture and grow in relationships? In whose terms is the ideal image of female adulthood chosen? This is a pivotal question for Ariel and becomes critical to me as her therapist as well.

As Ariel's therapist, I listen seriously to her needs. She needs me to listen to her, to recognize and respond to her as a real, caring person. She needs to know that I care about her. She wants my affection. She needs to have me acknowledge when she is right, and she needs me to admit when I am wrong. She does not want or need me to be perfect, and she does not want me to think or present myself as if I am. She does not want me to be defensive, or to force her to be on the defense. I ask myself, is Ariel right? Is she asking too much of me as her therapist? Do I feel inadequate in the face of her needs? And I ask myself, if this will free Ariel, if she is right, can I possibly free her from her pain by responding to her needs, in the structure of therapy?

I realized if I was going to be a good therapist to Ariel, I had to think deeply about how I practice, my model for therapy. This was scary for me, because I take her needs seriously, and I have to think about how I will respond to her in the context of my life, my children, my marriage, my needs and desires. Do I have room for Ariel in my life, as well as in my practice? When I listen personally to Ariel's requests to her parents, "listen to me, deal with me, trust me . . . ' I hear her also asking me to not create rigid molds and expectations that are clearly hierarchical and unpenetrable. She is asking me to challenge core structures of traditional psychodynamic therapy as I have been taught to practice it. In a funny way, I feel quite closely connected to Ariel through her request, because I realize that she is asking me, as a psychotherapist, to do the same thing that she, as a teenage girl, needs to learn to do. In this way our struggle is the same. Ariel and I both share a deeply intimate psychic struggle that comes from being female and trying to hold on to the truth and integrity of our experience within a culture, language and tradition comprised of structures that distort truths and experiences that don't fit.

As I work with Ariel and begin to address with her what feels right in the context of our work together, I watch myself think deeply about how I practice, and I see that some of my therapeutic responses and reactions to Ariel are counterintuitive to my training. If I look at the traditional model it feels wrong. Just as I believe that a therapy of adaptation is iatrogenic for girls with eating disorders, so too is a traditional model of psychotherapy. In order to respond to Ariel, I must challenge the order and mold of psychodynamic psychotherapy, and in so doing, model to her a way of resistance through which she could potentially "free" herself.

NAMING THE RELATIONSHIP

My struggle as a woman therapist writing about therapy in my own way is the same as the struggle that I must engage and support with my clients; that is, I have to fend off aspects of my training that would have me fit into traditionally defined ways of writing (like referring to myself in the third person as "the therapist") and practicing (like sitting on the couch together) that do not include or acknowledge aspects of my work that I believe to be essential and true and respectable.

For example, in spite of many significant differences between us (I have not struggled with an eating disorder, or with a family like hers, nor was I born post 1960's), I know my own struggle as a girl and an adult, a struggle to stay connected to myself and others, a struggle for my own voice. The themes of sorrow and loss, anger and alienation are familiar to me. I know my own version of them in myself, and I know them in my sisters, my mother, my women friends. And I know I can't function as a good therapist without thinking about my relationship to the girl in me. There are times when my immediate therapeutic response is a trustworthy response, but because it is counterintuitive to my training, I experience a silent struggle similar to the adolescent girl who wonders "Should I say what I think, or what I really think?" (Gilligan, 1990).

My practice is set up via an answering service. If clients want to reach me, they must go through a third party. There have been times when it made more emotional or relational sense for me to call Ariel rather than have her call my service and wait for a return call. A few times, I have given her my number and said call me at home. Each time, we go over what we'll do if it's not possible for me to speak, how I'll tell her. She needs to know that I will be honest with her about my availability. The first time Ariel calls me is hardly ideal for a working mother. It is one in the morning and she is sobbing. I had said to her, and I meant it, that if she is stirred up by what we have talked about during the session and she needs to talk at some other time, she should call me. In telling her that I don't expect her to fit her feelings into 50 minute segments, I am responding to her requests about not fitting into "molds, hierarchies, and treating her like a real person." Even though I know she may get me up, I have to go with what I feel will be healing for her, and I tell her that I hope I'm there when she calls. When I hear her crying voice, I go into another room and I tell her I'm getting my pillow and a blanket. I will not rush this or limit our time to ten minutes. I want her to know immediately that I welcome her call, even if it is in the middle of the night. I know what a big step it is for Ariel to reach out and call me in tears, and I feel the power of the moment for her and for our work together. After she has called, she is obviously worried when we meet again. I tell her how glad I was that she called, that she let herself. We go over her feelings about it, and mine. I laugh as I tell her that her assumption that I was probably up anyway is wrong. Even though calling me at home is disruptive, and not something I wish to do regularly, I believe it is an essential step for Ariel to get well.

Another time Ariel is intensely worried about an encounter with a peer at school. We discuss the nuances of the conflict between them, and talk about what Ariel wants to say. I know this is a moment of great importance for her, and I decide to say "I'll call you around four to find out how it went." I know this is contrary to standard techniques of wait and see how she brings it up, if she does, etc. I tell her I will call her because it makes emotional and therapeutic sense to me. I am the one who wants to hear at that time, and it is easier for me to call her. Also, I want her to know and experience that I think about her and care about her outside of our time limit. My reasons for doing this are several, and combined, feel necessary for her therapy and my involvement in my work. Ariel really matters to me, and so does my work with her, and I will challenge the mold of therapy if it is necessary for her recovery. It is clear to me that we need to create a way of being together where she doesn't feel that she is asking too much, where she can be herself and so can I.

Rather than always respond to Ariel by asking her what she

thinks and feels ("how do you feel about that"), there are moments when I tell Ariel directly how what she is saying affects me. Ariel has told me that she needs to be treated "like a real person," in a real relationship. I believe that in order for her to feel related to as a real person, she needs to hear directly from me how what she says affects me, influences me. I want her to experience in therapy, a relationship where it is very clear that I am present and moved by what she is saying, and that what she says counts. I have said to Ariel. "I hate that this happened to you," "I'm so sad to hear this" or "your telling me this makes my day." When I am wrong about something, I tell her. When I see her shining, I tell her. And when she asks, and it is true, I tell her, "Of course I love you,"[1] I have also said to her, "therapy is a completely weird relationship," and together we have at several times gone over the structure of therapy critiqing it together, acknowledging its oddities together. To not do this would be to superimpose another mold on Ariel and make her feel defective for not fitting into it with ease (see Steiner-Adair, 1990). In so doing, I would collude with the very message that is so devastating for Ariel, that she must learn to take a stand apart from and challenge.

My job is to create, nurture and sustain a relationship with Ariel in which she can constantly "refine the truths" she tells herself and others (Rich, 1979). I see therapy as a process of going deeper and deeper into the layers of oneself in order to discover how one got to this point of pain. This room becomes a sanctuary, a resting place, where a kind of slow learning occurs. I know that there are things I know about the phenomenon of eating disorders, and psychic pain which manifests itself in numerous ways, and I can teach her a lot that will bring Ariel back to herself. I also trust that Ariel already knows things she needs to know in order to get better, and my job is to help her uncover what she knows. I pay close attention to her need to define our space. Early on in our meetings she says "I hate these chairs. Can we sit on the couch?" "Sure," I say, "I'd like that." Together we overthrow another structure, literally and metaphorically. She kicks off her shoes and I do the same. This has become our joining ritual, the shedding of the shoes, the foot soldier's gear. Over time we come to share a blanket over our toes. She tells me her feet stink and I tell her I don't care. Time after time she hears me say, "I don't care about all the things that others would say are bad or smelly about you." Sometimes when she's crying, I reach out and hold her foot, put my hand on her leg, constantly asking myself to challenge the rules in order to be connected in the way that feels necessary, safe and emotionally right to me. These are difficult moments, because my instincts and my thinking from my feminist framework is counter to some of my clinical training.

When I work with Ariel, I often experience therapy as a kind of teaching. This is an arduous task initially, because Ariel has gotten so used to using binging and purging to numb herself and to flee from herself, because there has been no safe place where it isn't dangerous for her to know what she already knows. Her parents have tried to make it safe for Ariel to speak about her perceptions; they have tried. But they have been unsuccessful for reasons Ariel and I will discover. Because Ariel has struggled for so many years protecting others and herself from her perceptions, some of them are confused and out of perspective. At her worst, Ariel dissociates from herself when she can not tolerate the anxiety of knowing what she knows or her confusion about what she doesn't understand, and one of my early tasks is to teach her to stay in her body and in her self and learn to feel again what seems intolerable to feel.

It doesn't take long to get Ariel rolling gently back into herself. Sometimes the waves of remembering are rough and she thrashes – "I hate this, I hate them. I hate that this is how my life has been." Sometimes the waves are steady streams of tears, as we sit on the couch and she softly cries, our feet overlapping. I encourage Ariel over and over to trust the rhythms of her remembering, and together we go through a time of her mourning. This is a sad time for Ariel, but it is not one of endless sorrow; in the process of naming her pain she frees herself from unconsciously embodying her pain. At the end of this time, she brings me her favorite pictures of herself. She is eight years old, standing by a tree. She says "I love this girl that I was. I was so innocent then. It's so sad I had to grow up and leave her behind" (see also Hancock, 1989). I am flooded by the sweetness in her wide open eyes. Like Ariel, I too wish she could have found a way to grow up and keep that little girl central to her self. Ariel describes this time in her life as "The last time I could be myself, before things got so complicated and there were so many expectations on me that I couldn't handle, that weren't me." We talk about what it means to grow up.

When I am doing therapy, I often remember individuals who helped me at different junctures in my life, who by their very presence, introduced and infused me with a positive experience of being a woman and the community of women. Women who helped me see ways I could make the leap from here to there, from this age or place to the next. I had the extreme good fortune to attend an excellent girls' camp and I often think of the director of this camp in this way. She lives in me as my first experience of the wise woman. Her aging mother who founded the camp, read us *The Little Prince* (St. Exupery, 1943) and other classics on rainy days, and her mother died one summer at camp. I remember her dying at camp vividly, a peaceful death that was gently and gracefully and certainly positively experienced by me. She was, I believe, eighty five and I was fourteen, her daughter fifty four, her daughter-in-law twenty nine. This was one of tho first deaths in my life and I am grateful to have been in the company of these women, who each in her own way introduced me to dying as a part of life. There have been and continue to be women in my life who have made an abiding difference in my development, enabling me to become who I am. And I have in my office, high up in a corner shelf always looking at me, an apple doll of a gardening granny (given to me by my husband when I was missing my maternal grandmother who was an endless source of support and enthusiasm for me) and I often look to this image to remind me of the patience required to tend to growth and development, whether it's the seasons outdoors or the inner timetable of an individual.

In conjunction with her discovery about her eating disorder, I want to teach Ariel my understanding of the values of wholeness, affirmation of the natural body, and the wisdom of nature. I also believe that the more Ariel becomes comfortable with her intensity, her passions, her desires, her furies with me, her rage, the better able she will be to be herself and speak from these parts of herself in her life. I see therapy as a process of careful listening and responding, dancing to inner rhythms in her that are both confluent and discordant with the world around her. Our task is to better understand Ariel's relationship to her self, her body, others and the world, and I listen carefully for repeating themes.

Throughout our work, we talk about menstruation, defloration, conception, pregnancy, birth, nursing, mothering, menopause, aging, death – the ordinary work of women's lives. We talk about the metaphorical meaning of these natural phases, and in so doing, a feminine pattern of identity (Kubler-Merrill, 1990). I tell her stories about the connection between the lunar cycle and women's cycle. We talk about the light and the dark phases of the moon and her moods, the light and the darkness in herself that are both necessary and acceptable parts of the human and natural order.

We talk about love and true love and her vision of right relationships. We talk about meanness, evil, anger, jealousy, envy, intimidation, poverty, physical and sexual violence. A lot of therapy time is intermittently spent discussing relationships and what is the right thing to do based on how she truly feels. I listen to her describe her friends and her worries about misses and failures in relationships: "I didn't know what to say. . . no idea what I felt . . . I just don't know . . . I was speechless . . . I couldn't speak . . . I was dying to talk, he wasn't listening . . . it was so unfair because he hadn't heard what I said . . . I hate it when she doesn't ask me what I think. . , I was scared to death to tell . . . " And I feel her excitement when she speaks in the language of corrections in connections: "really there, really listened, truly felt, really got me, awesome sweet."

I want to teach Ariel to learn to tune into her silences, wait with herself, until she comes to herself in sensation, feeling or thought, to challenge the mold that is about speed and always knowing in a competitive or superficial way. We talk about how the binge keeps her from herself. She is afraid to be with herself. I talk with her and model with her the value of slowness, the concept of pace, so opposite from the fast world she and I live in. "How do you use silence Ariel?" I want her to discover in herself the companion of quiet compassionate listening, with me, and ultimately, with herself. Her journal becomes her ears for herself. There is an annihilating silence in her when she fights herself – but there is also a healing silence in her, a creative silence that will birth her writing, her victories of voice, and her healing process. Just as there is a silence that destroys, there is a silence that creates and heals. Like Woolf's (1929) room of one's own, she needs a place to contemplate, to receive herself – I remember her early dismissals, "this is so weird" "This is so weird, this is so different for you," I say, "to be in a space that is dedicated to you finding out who you are with no blame, no judgment" with receptive listening, gestation, time after time. Quiet time, and then comes more, re-membering. Over time, the dis-membering ceases.

MAKING A NEW ORDER

Two years later, Ariel's recovery is still on-going. She is symptom free, no longer binging or purging, no longer morose, depressed or suicidal, no longer excessively exercising or overly preoccupied with her weight. Sometimes she still feels she is overweight, but she is willing to live with it in exchange for not binging. Sometimes she still doesn't like how she looks, but not as intensely: I think it's safe to say she likes enough other things about herself so that her appearance isn't as central an issue. She is doing well in school, which matters to her, has good friends and a very sweet, very loving relationship with a young man (something she thought was impossible). She continues to write in her journal, and she is writing a novel about a family. She is far more outspoken about herself than previously. And although she still struggles with the risks of speaking out, she struggles directly in herself, and she feels able to make choices previously invisible to her. She is more direct with her parents, and their relationship has changed in some ways, remarkably. Her room is more often than not, neat. The day Ariel cleaned up her room for the first time in well over six months was a signal event in therapy. Finally she could see a way to create a new order in her life, a different order, her own order. She understands that her room gets messy when she gets confused and can no longer see a way to fit herself into "the bureau drawers of society."

Ultimately, I must say that I do not see an easy solution to Ariel's dilemma in the world as it is now. Her conflict is internal, but it mirrors external impasses, both in the culture and in models of therapy. For myself, the only solution I have found to function as a woman therapist working with teenagers with eating disorders is to uncover and dismantle the false facades of therapy at the same time as help girls with eating disorders uncover and dismantle the false facades of the world they are unable to inhabit. In this way our struggles are mutual, and reciprocally connected to each other. In this challenge, we meet as two females, each in our individual lives struggling to reveal and challenge molds that are disabling, whether developmentally or professionally. Herein Ariel and I are deeply connected to each other as we work very hard, together and separately, to hold on to the healthy voice of resistance in each of us, and to find people in our lives who will "go that hard way with us" (Rich, 1979).

ENDNOTES

1. Some therapists routinely avoid statements like this, and others will make them ordinarily when there is a common and safe meaning that is shared between client and therapist. In this instance, I had good reason to believe that we were both clear in understanding my statement to mean "of course I care about you and am committed to you." Ariel and I talked about many different kinds of love and attachment, and that there are different kinds of love.

2. In addition to Ariel's individual therapy with me, she was also seen for a period of time by a clinical nutritionist, and her parents were in therapy as well. There were a few occasions when I saw Ariel with her parents, and when I participated in the couples therapy.

REFERENCES

Boskind-Lodahl, M. (1976). Cinderella's step-sisters: A feminist perspective on anorexia and bulimia. *Signs: Journal of women in culture and society.* 2,324-356.

Gilligan, C. (1990). Teaching Shakespeare's Sisters: Notes from the underground of female adolescence. In C. Gilligan, N. Lyons, T. Hanmer (Eds.), *Making connections: The relational worlds of adolescent girls at the Emma Willard School.* Cambridge MA: Harvard University Press.

Gilligan, C. (1989). Joining the resistance: Psychology, politics, girls and women. *Michigan Quarterly Review, 29*,4,501-536.

Hancock, E. (1989). *The Girl Within.* New York: E. P. Dutton.

Kubler-Merrill, A. (1990). *Notes from the women's self analytic study group.* Unpublished manuscript, St. George, ME. paper.

Miller, J. (1984). The development of women's sense of self. *Work in progress,* No. 12. Wellsley MA: Stone Center Working Papers Series.

Rich, A. (1979). *On lies, secrets, and silence.* New York: Norton p. 188.

Steiner-Adair, C.(1986). The body politic: Normal female adolescent development and the development of eating disorders. *Journal of the American Academy of Psychoanalysis, 14*,95-114.

Steiner-Adair, C. (1989). Educating the voice of the wise woman: College students and bulimia. In L. Whitaker & W. Davis (Eds.), *The Bulimic college student: Evaluation, treatment, and prevention.* New York: The Haworth Press, Inc.

Steiner-Adair, C. (1990). New maps of development, new models of therapy: The psychology of women and the treatment of eating disorders. In C. Johnson (Ed.), *Psychodynamic treatment of anorexia nervosa and bulimia.* New York: Guilford.

St. Exupery, A. (1943). *The little prince.* New York: Harcourt Brace.

Surrey, J. (1985). Self in relation: A theory of women's development. *Work in progress No. 14.* Wellsley MA: Stone Center Working Paper Series.

Wooley, S., Wooley, O., & Dryenforth, S. (1979). Obesity and women: A neglected feminist topic. *Women Studies International Quarterly,* 2, 81-92.

Woolf, V. (1929) *A room of one's own.* New York: Harcourt Brace.

Index

